WITHDRAWN

Carnegie Mellon

MEDICARE: A PRIMER

HEALTH CARE ISSUES, COSTS AND ACCESS SERIES

The Health Care Financial Crisis: Strategies for Overcoming an "Unholy Trinity"
Cal Clark and Rene McEldowney (Editors)
2001. ISBN: 1-56072-924-4

Health Care Crisis in America
James B. Prince (Editor)
2006. ISBN: 1-59454-698-4

**A New Epidemic: Harm in Health Care-How to Make Rational Decisions about
Medical and Surgical Treatment**
Aage R. Moller
2007. ISBN: 1-60021-884-9

Decision Making in Medicine and Health Care
Partricia C. Tolana (Editor)
2008. ISBN: 1-60021-870-9

Decision Making in Medicine and Health Care
Partricia C. Tolana (Editor)
2008. ISBN: 978-1-60692-561-4 (Online Book)

Social Sciences in Health Care and Medicine
Janet B. Garner and Thelma C. Christiansen (Editors)
2008. ISBN: 978-1-60456-286-6

Health Care Policies
Linda A. Bartlette and Ida F. Lawson (Editors)
2008. ISBN: 978-1-60456-352-8

Handbook of Stress and Burnout in Health Care
Jonathon R.B. Halbesleben (Editor)
2008. ISBN: 978-1-60456-500-3

Health Care Costs: Outlook and Options
Raymond W. Inhurst (Editor)
2009. ISBN: 978-1-60692-151-7

Medicare Payment Policies to Physicians
Katherine V. Bergen (Editor)
2009. ISBN: 978-1-60692-131-4

Comparative Effectiveness of Medical Treatments
Peter Villa and Sophia Brun
2009 ISBN: 978-1-60741-109-3 (Softcover)

Health Care Costs: Causes, Effects and Control
Bernice R. Hofmann (Editor)
2009. ISBN: 978-1-60456-976-6

A Guide to Public Health Research Needs
Raymond I. Turner
2009. ISBN: 978-1-60692-852-3

A Guide to Public Health Research Needs
Raymond I. Turner
2009. ISBN: 978-1-60876-605-5 (Online Book)

Handbook of Dental Care: Diagnostic, Preventative and Restorative Services
Jose C. Taggart (Editor)
2009. ISBN: 978-1-60741-281-6

Generic Drugs: Needs and Issues
Ryan S. Blanton (Editor)
2009. ISBN: 978-1-60692-843-1

Medicare: A Primer
Alice R. Williamson (Editor)
2009. ISBN: 978-1-60741-108-6

HEALTH CARE ISSUES, COSTS AND ACCESS SERIES

MEDICARE: A PRIMER

Alice R. Williamson
Editor

Nova Science Publishers, Inc.
New York

NOTICE TO THE READER

The Publisher has taken reasonable care in the preparation of this book, but makes no expressed or implied warranty of any kind and assumes no responsibility for any errors or omissions. No liability is assumed for incidental or consequential damages in connection with or arising out of information contained in this book. The Publisher shall not be liable for any special, consequential, or exemplary damages resulting, in whole or in part, from the readers' use of, or reliance upon, this material. Any parts of this book based on government reports are so indicated and copyright is claimed for those parts to the extent applicable to compilations of such works.

Independent verification should be sought for any data, advice or recommendations contained in this book. In addition, no responsibility is assumed by the publisher for any injury and/or damage to persons or property arising from any methods, products, instructions, ideas or otherwise contained in this publication.

This publication is designed to provide accurate and authoritative information with regard to the subject matter covered herein. It is sold with the clear understanding that the Publisher is not engaged in rendering legal or any other professional services. If legal or any other expert assistance is required, the services of a competent person should be sought. FROM A DECLARATION OF PARTICIPANTS JOINTLY ADOPTED BY A COMMITTEE OF THE AMERICAN BAR ASSOCIATION AND A COMMITTEE OF PUBLISHERS.

LIBRARY OF CONGRESS CATALOGING-IN-PUBLICATION DATA

Medicare : a primer / editor, Alice R. Williamson.
   p. ; cm.
 Includes index.
 Chapters published separately in print and online.
 ISBN 978-1-60741-108-6 (hardcover)·
1. Medicare. I. Williamson, Alice R.
 [DNLM: 1. Medicare--Collected Works. WT 31 M4852 2009]
 RA412.3.M4266 2009
 368.4'2600973--dc22
                              2009027739

Published by Nova Science Publishers, Inc. ✦ *New York*

CONTENTS

Preface   vii

Chapter 1   The Impact of Medicare's Payment Rates on the Volume
             of Services Provided by Skilled Nursing Facilities   1
             Congressional Budget Office

Chapter 2   Factors Underlying the Growth in Medicare's Spending
             for Physician's Services   25
             Congressional Budget Office

Chapter 3   Improving Medicare Efficiency and Value   53
             Medicare Payment Advisory Commission

Chapter 4   Medicare: A Primer   69
             Jennifer O'Sullivan

Chapter Sources   107

Index   109

PREFACE

Congress continues to register concern about the rapid rise in Medicare spending and the ability of existing funding mechanisms to support the program over the longterm. A combination of factors has contributed to the rapid increase in Medicare costs. These include increases in overall medical costs, advances in health care delivery and medical technology, the aging of the population, and longer life spans. The issues confronting the program are not new; nor are the possible solutions likely to get any easier. For a number of years, various options have been suggested; however, legislative changes have focused on short-term issues. There is no consensus on the long-term approach that should be taken. This book provides an overview of Medicare. It begins with a brief program history, and then outlines the key features of Parts A and B, also known as "Original Medicare." That is followed by overviews of Part C and Part D, a discussion of program financing, and a brief discussion of future program directions. It will be updated to reflect any legislative changes.

Chapter 1 - The central long-term fiscal challenge facing the nation involves rising costs in Medicare, Medicaid, and other federal health-related programs. The Congressional Budget Office (CBO) is therefore expanding its work in examining the rising costs within the nation's federal health programs as well as possible policy responses.

Medicare's benefit package includes coverage for short-term posthospitalization care in skilled nursing facilities (SNFs). Medicare beneficiaries can qualify to receive Medicare-covered SNF care if they previously had an inpatient hospital stay of at least three days and if they require skilled nursing services. SNFs' covered services include rehabilitation and medical services such as intravenous drug therapy.

Medicare spent $19.5 billion on SNF care in 2006, which is about 6.6 percent of total Medicare spending in the fee-for-service sector.[1] The system Medicare uses to determine SNF payment rates has undergone several major revisions in the past decade, the most significant of which was the introduction of a prospective payment system (PPS) in 1998. Under that system, Medicare pays a daily rate for SNF care that is calculated by combining a national base rate, a local wage index adjustor, and a case-mix adjustor. In the years since the PPS was implemented, payment rates have been changed repeatedly, with the impact of those changes varying substantially across SNFs.

This Congressional Budget Office background paper measures how the volume of Medicare-covered SNF services adjusts in response to changes in Medicare's SNF payment rates (the so-called volume response). The payment rate equals the payment received by a medical provider in exchange for providing a single unit of medical service; that rate comprises payments both from Medicare and from the patient. Although Medicare's payment rates for SNFs have been changed repeatedly over the past decade, beneficiaries' coinsurance for SNF care and other factors that affect the demand for that care have remained relatively stable. The volume response measured in this paper, therefore, reflects mainly a supply-driven phenomenon.

This paper includes two separate analyses. The two analyses take similar approaches, but they measure changes in payment rates and volume using different units of analysis over different periods. The use of two separate analyses provides a robustness check and offers some evidence on the sensitivity of the key findings to the analytical approach taken. In the geographic-level analysis, changes from 1997 to 2001 in SNF volume and payment rates are measured for 3,436 different hospital service areas, or HSAs. (HSAs are geographic areas corresponding to local health care markets.) The years 1997 and 2001 were chosen for the geographic analysis because they fall on either side of the implementation of the SNF prospective payment system. In the provider-level analysis, year-to-year changes in SNF volume and payment rates are measured for each SNF from 1999 through 2003. During those years, there were several legislative changes to Medicare's SNF payment rates under the PPS.

Although most SNFs operate as units within freestanding nursing facilities, a significant share of SNFs are hospital based. Freestanding and hospital-based SNFs differ in several important ways. At the median, Medicare-covered SNF days made up 11 percent of total patient days in freestanding facilities in 2005 (the remaining patients in freestanding SNFs are non-Medicare patients or long-term care residents).[2] On average, hospital-based SNFs tend to largely serve Medicare beneficiaries. To account for that and other differences, this analysis measures volume responses among freestanding and hospital-based SNFs separately.

The geographic-level and provider-level analyses together provide evidence that the volume of Medicare-covered SNF days varies positively with Medicare's SNF payment rates. For example, a change of 1 percent in Medicare's payment rate for SNFs is estimated to result in a modest change of 0.13 percent in volume (based on the geographic-level analysis) or 0.23 percent (based on the provider-level analysis), with volume changing in the same direction as payment rates. In both the geographic-level and provider-level analyses, that same direction of volume response is found among hospital-based and freestanding SNFs.

The geographic-level analysis suggests that SNFs increase the volume of services they provide in response to an increase in payment rates and likewise decrease volume in response to a decrease in payment rates, with the magnitude of those responses being roughly similar. The provider-level analysis also suggests a modest and statistically significant increase in the volume of SNF services in response to payment increases (in that analysis, the response to payment decreases was not statistically significant). Overall, those findings imply that the impact on Medicare's spending of a change in Medicare's SNF payment rates will be magnified to some extent by the volume response, meaning that an increase in payment rates will lead to a somewhat larger percentage increase in Medicare's spending on skilled nursing facilities. The central long-term fiscal challenge facing the nation involves rising costs in Medicare, Medicaid, and other federal health-related programs. The Congressional Budget Office (CBO) is therefore expanding its work in examining the rising costs within the nation's federal health programs as well as possible policy responses. One rapidly growing component of Medicare involves payments for physicians' services, which is the focus of this paper.

Medicare compensates physicians for services they provide under the Supplemental Medical Insurance program, or Medicare Part B, on the basis of a fee schedule that specifies payment rates for each type of covered service. Payment rates are calculated in three steps:

First, the fee schedule stipulates relative value units (RVUs), which measure the resources required to provide a given service. Second, payments are adjusted to account for geographical differences in input prices. Third, a "conversion factor" translates the geographically adjusted RVUs for a particular service into a dollar amount.

Annual updates to payment rates are governed by a mechanism known as the Sustainable Growth Rate (SGR), which aims to control Medicare's outlays for physicians' services.[1] Established in the Balanced Budget Act of 1997 (Public Law 105-33) and implemented in 1998, the SGR formula operates by setting a target amount for such expenditures and adjusting payment rates to reflect differences between actual spending and spending targets (both of which are measured on an annual and a cumulative basis). If actual spending under the SGR does not deviate from the expenditure targets, payment rates under the physician fee schedule are simply increased by the percentage change in the Medicare economic index, or MEI. However, if actual spending is above the targets set by the SGR formula, the update to payment rates will be smaller than the increase in the MEI. If spending is below the targets, the update will be higher than the increase in the MEI. Those adjustments are designed so that, over a period of several years, cumulative spending will be brought into line with the cumulative expenditure target.

Annual updates to payment rates for physicians' services have varied widely in recent years, ranging from a minimum of about -5 percent (in 1999 and in 2002) to a maximum of roughly 5 percent (in 2000). (When adjusted to account for changes in the MEI, updates to payment rates have ranged from about -8 percent to 3 percent.) According to CBO's estimates, if provisions of current law remained unchanged, Medicare's payments to physicians would be reduced by about 10 percent in 2008 and by about 5 percent annually over the following several years. However, because lawmakers overrode the SGR mechanism between 2003 and 2007—replacing negative updates with small positive or zero updates—it is uncertain whether the SGR mechanism will be allowed to operate as specified.

Although updates to Medicare's payment rates have fluctuated since the SGR was established, spending for physicians' services under the fee schedule has increased steadily, rising by 79.2 percent between 1997 and 2005. Even after adjusting for changes in the cost of providing physicians' services—as measured by the Medicare economic index—and for growth in the number of beneficiaries enrolled in the program, spending on physicians' services has increased by 34.5 percent.[3]

Chapter 2 - The central long-term fiscal challenge facing the nation involves rising costs in Medicare, Medicaid, and other federal health-related programs. The Congressional Budget Office (CBO) is therefore expanding its work in examining the rising costs within the nation's federal health programs as well as possible policy responses. One rapidly growing component of Medicare involves payments for physicians' services, which is the focus of this paper.

Medicare compensates physicians for services they provide under the Supplemental Medical Insurance program, or Medicare Part B, on the basis of a fee schedule that specifies payment rates for each type of covered service. Payment rates are calculated in three steps: First, the fee schedule stipulates relative value units (RVUs), which measure the resources required to provide a given service. Second, payments are adjusted to account for geographical differences in input prices. Third, a "conversion factor" translates the geographically adjusted RVUs for a particular service into a dollar amount.

Annual updates to payment rates are governed by a mechanism known as the Sustainable Growth Rate (SGR), which aims to control Medicare's outlays for physicians' services.[1] Established in the Balanced Budget Act of 1997 (Public Law 105-33) and implemented in 1998, the SGR formula operates by setting a target amount for such expenditures and adjusting payment rates to reflect differences between actual spending and spending targets (both of which are measured on an annual and a cumulative basis). If actual spending under the SGR does not deviate from the expenditure targets, payment rates under the physician fee schedule are simply increased by the percentage change in the Medicare economic index, or MEI.[2] However, if actual spending is above the targets set by the SGR formula, the update to payment rates will be smaller than the increase in the MEI. If spending is below the targets, the update will be higher than the increase in the MEI. Those adjustments are designed so that, over a period of several years, cumulative spending will be brought into line with the cumulative expenditure target.

Annual updates to payment rates for physicians' services have varied widely in recent years, ranging from a minimum of about -5 percent (in 1999 and in 2002) to a maximum of roughly 5 percent (in 2000). (When adjusted to account for changes in the MEI, updates to payment rates have ranged from about -8 percent to 3 percent.) According to CBO's estimates, if provisions of current law remained unchanged, Medicare's payments to physicians would be reduced by about 10 percent in 2008 and by about 5 percent annually over the following several years. However, because lawmakers overrode the SGR mechanism between 2003 and 2007—replacing negative updates with small positive or zero updates—it is uncertain whether the SGR mechanism will be allowed to operate as specified.

Although updates to Medicare's payment rates have fluctuated since the SGR was established, spending for physicians' services under the fee schedule has increased steadily, rising by 79.2 percent between 1997 and 2005. Even after adjusting for changes in the cost of providing physicians' services—as measured by the Medicare economic index—and for growth in the number of beneficiaries enrolled in the program, spending on physicians' services has increased by 34.5 percent.

Chapter 3 - There is currently a great deal of interest in improving the efficiency of the Medicare program. This interest is driven not only by the desire to make Medicare a better program but also by growing concern about the sustainability of Medicare spending. Medicare as a public payer has suffered from the same persistently high growth in health care cost that has plagued all sectors of the health financing community. Medicare spending grew 9.3 percent annually between 1980 and 2004, on average, considerably higher than the average annual rate of growth in gross domestic product (GDP) of 6.5 percent for that same period. While growth in GDP—the measure of goods and services produced in the United States—is used as a benchmark of how much additional growth in expenditure society can afford, other measures illustrate the more direct impacts of growth in Medicare spending on the program's beneficiaries. Between 1970 and 2005, the average monthly Social Security benefit increased by an inflation-adjusted average annual rate of 1.6 percent; during the same period, Medicare Supplementary Medical Insurance premiums grew by more than 4 percent annually. Recent Part B premium increases have offset 30 percent to 40 percent of the dollar increase in the average Social Security benefit. Yet, despite this rapid growth in spending, a large body of evidence suggests the increased cost of health care has not come with a corresponding increase in quality. The Institute of Medicine, in its 2001 report *Crossing the Quality Chasm*, suggested that while care may be improving in many settings, significant gaps remain between what is known to be good care and the care delivered, and it is still all too common for beneficiaries not to receive high-quality health care.

Chapter 4 - Medicare is the nation's health insurance program for persons aged 65 and over and certain disabled persons. In FY2008, the program will cover an estimated 44.6 million persons (37.4 million aged and 7.3 million disabled) at a total cost of $459.4 billion. Federal costs (after deduction of beneficiary premiums and other offsetting receipts) will total $389.9 billion. In FY2008, federal Medicare spending will represent approximately 13% of the total federal budget and 3% of GDP. Medicare is an entitlement program, which means that it is required to pay for services provided to eligible persons, so long as specific criteria are met.

Since Medicare was enacted in 1965, it has undergone considerable changes. First, program coverage was expanded to include the disabled and persons with endstage renal disease (ESRD). Over time, increasing attention was placed on stemming the rapid increase in program spending, which outpaced projections, even in the initial years. This was typically achieved through tightening rules governing payments to providers of services and stemming the annual updates in such payments. The program moved from payments based on "reasonable costs" and "reasonable charges" to payment systems under which a pre-determined payment amount is established for a specified unit of service. At the same time, beneficiaries were given the option to obtain covered services through private managed care arrangements. Most Medicare payment provisions were incorporated into larger budget reconciliation bills designed to control overall federal spending.

In 2003, Congress enacted a major Medicare bill, the Medicare Prescription Drug, Improvement, and Modernization Act of 2003 (MMA). This legislation placed increasing emphasis on private sector management of benefits. It also created a new voluntary outpatient prescription drug benefit to be administered by private entities. Further, it introduced the concept of means testing into what had previously been strictly a social insurance program.

Congress continues to register concern about the rapid rise in Medicare spending and the ability of existing funding mechanisms to support the program over the longterm. A combination of factors has contributed to the rapid increase in Medicare costs. These include increases in overall medical costs, advances in health care delivery and medical technology, the aging of the population, and longer life spans. The issues confronting the program are not new; nor are the possible solutions likely to get any easier. For a number of years, various options have been suggested; however, legislative changes have focused on short-term issues. There is no consensus on the long-term approach that should be taken.

This report provides an overview of Medicare. It begins with a brief program history, and then outlines the key features of Parts A and B, also known as "Original Medicare." That is followed by overviews of Part C and Part D, a discussion of program financing, and a brief discussion of future program directions. It will be updated to reflect any legislative changes.

In: Medicare: A Primer
Editor: Alice R. Williamson

ISBN: 978-1-60741-108-6
© 2009 Nova Science Publishers, Inc.

Chapter 1

THE IMPACT OF MEDICARE'S PAYMENT RATES ON THE VOLUME OF SERVICES PROVIDED BY SKILLED NURSING FACILITIES

United States Congressional Budget Office

SUMMARY AND INTRODUCTION

The central long-term fiscal challenge facing the nation involves rising costs in Medicare, Medicaid, and other federal health-related programs. The Congressional Budget Office (CBO) is therefore expanding its work in examining the rising costs within the nation's federal health programs as well as possible policy responses.

Medicare's benefit package includes coverage for short-term posthospitalization care in skilled nursing facilities (SNFs). Medicare beneficiaries can qualify to receive Medicare-covered SNF care if they previously had an inpatient hospital stay of at least three days and if they require skilled nursing services. SNFs' covered services include rehabilitation and medical services such as intravenous drug therapy.

Medicare spent $19.5 billion on SNF care in 2006, which is about 6.6 percent of total Medicare spending in the fee-for-service sector.[1] The system Medicare uses to determine SNF payment rates has undergone several major revisions in the past decade, the most significant of which was the introduction of a prospective payment system (PPS) in 1998. Under that system, Medicare pays a daily rate for SNF care that is calculated by combining a national base rate, a local wage index adjustor, and a case-mix adjustor. In the years since the PPS was implemented, payment rates have been changed repeatedly, with the impact of those changes varying substantially across SNFs.

This Congressional Budget Office background paper measures how the volume of Medicare-covered SNF services adjusts in response to changes in Medicare's SNF payment rates (the so-called volume response). The payment rate equals the payment received by a medical provider in exchange for providing a single unit of medical service; that rate comprises payments both from Medicare and from the patient. Although Medicare's payment rates for SNFs have been changed repeatedly over the past decade, beneficiaries' coinsurance for SNF care and other factors that affect the demand for that care have remained relatively stable. The volume response measured in this paper, therefore, reflects mainly a supply-driven phenomenon.

This paper includes two separate analyses. The two analyses take similar approaches, but they measure changes in payment rates and volume using different units of analysis over different periods. The use of two separate analyses provides a robustness check and offers some evidence on the sensitivity of the key findings to the analytical approach taken. In the geographic-level analysis, changes from 1997 to 2001 in SNF volume and payment rates are measured for 3,436 different hospital service areas, or HSAs. (HSAs are geographic areas corresponding to local health care markets.) The years 1997 and 2001 were chosen for the geographic analysis because they fall on either side of the implementation of the SNF prospective payment system. In the provider-level analysis, year-to-year changes in SNF volume and payment rates are measured for each SNF from 1999 through 2003. During those years, there were several legislative changes to Medicare's SNF payment rates under the PPS.

Although most SNFs operate as units within freestanding nursing facilities, a significant share of SNFs are hospital based. Freestanding and hospital-based SNFs differ in several important ways. At the median, Medicare-covered SNF days made up 11 percent of total patient days in freestanding facilities in 2005 (the remaining patients in freestanding SNFs are non-Medicare patients or long-term care residents).[2] On average, hospital-based SNFs tend to largely serve Medicare beneficiaries. To account for that and other differences, this analysis measures volume responses among freestanding and hospital-based SNFs separately.

The geographic-level and provider-level analyses together provide evidence that the volume of Medicare-covered SNF days varies positively with Medicare's SNF payment rates. For example, a change of 1 percent in Medicare's payment rate for SNFs is estimated to result in a modest change of 0.13 percent in volume (based on the geographic-level analysis) or 0.23 percent (based on the provider-level analysis), with volume changing in the same direction as payment rates. In both the geographic-level and provider-level analyses, that same direction of volume response is found among hospital-based and freestanding SNFs.

The geographic-level analysis suggests that SNFs increase the volume of services they provide in response to an increase in payment rates and likewise decrease volume in response to a decrease in payment rates, with the magnitude of those responses being roughly similar. The provider-level analysis also suggests a modest and statistically significant increase in the volume of SNF services in response to payment increases (in that analysis, the response to payment decreases was not statistically significant). Overall, those findings imply that the impact on Medicare's spending of a change in Medicare's SNF payment rates will be magnified to some extent by the volume response, meaning that an increase in payment rates will lead to a somewhat larger percentage increase in Medicare's spending on skilled nursing facilities.

BACKGROUND INFORMATION

Volume response refers to a change in the volume of medical services in response to a change in the payment rate that medical providers receive. The measurement of volume response is relevant to CBO's estimates of the impact on Medicare's spending of proposed changes in Medicare's payment rates. For example, a proposed increase of 1 percent in Medicare's payment rates for SNFs could increase Medicare's spending on that care by more than 1 percent if volume increased as a result of the change in payment rates, or by less than 1 percent if volume decreased.[3] To date, there has been little research on changes in Medicare's payment rates for skilled nursing facilities and how they affect Medicare's spending.

In theory, providers will respond in certain ways to changes in payment rates. This section of the paper examines providers' responses and reviews the relevant empirical research. It also looks at Medicare's payment system for SNFs and the payment changes that underlie the analyses in this paper.

The Volume Response: A Theoretical Framework

In general, a change in the volume of medical services provided in response to a given change in the payment rate may stem from supply-side factors, demand-side factors, or both. An example of a demand-side volume response would be a coinsurance arrangement in which beneficiaries' out-of-pocket payment equals a fixed share of the payment rate. Changes in the payment rate would lead directly to changes in the out-of-pocket payment, which would affect beneficiaries' demand for services. In the case of Medicare's SNF services, however, the out-ofpocket payment does not vary with the payment rate.

For the first 20 days of a SNF stay, Medicare beneficiaries face no cost sharing for SNF care. Beginning on the 21st day of a SNF stay, Medicare beneficiaries pay a daily coinsurance amount. In recent years, that amount has increased roughly in line with general inflation, rising from $95 in 1997 to $119 in 2007. The out-of-pocket payment for Medicare's SNF services does not vary across types of services, across the facilities themselves, or across regions, and it has remained stable over time. That fact implies that changes in SNF volume in response to changes in Medicare's payment rate mainly reflect changes in the supply or availability of SNF care (which depends on factors such as input prices and licensing requirements) rather than changes in the demand for SNF care (which depends on factors such as beneficiaries' coinsurance, health status, and income).

Most previous research on the volume response of health care providers has focused on physicians. The behavior of physicians has been analyzed as a labor-supply decision, with a trade-off between working longer hours and earning more income or having more leisure time and earning less income.[4] An increase in fees paid to physicians will, according to the standard theoretical model, have two supply-side effects, which work in opposite directions. First, physicians will substitute work for leisure time because working has become more financially rewarding; second, physicians will decrease their supply of labor (work hours) because their potential income has increased and they can afford to "buy" more leisure time ("potential income" equals the amount a physician could earn if he or she only worked and spent no time on leisure activities).

In the case of Medicare's payments to physicians, changes in physicians' fees also have a demand-side effect because of Medicare's cost-sharing arrangements. Medicare beneficiaries' cost sharing for physicians' services is set equal to a percentage of the physicians' fees. (Different approaches are used to determine beneficiaries' cost sharing for SNF care and for other nonphysician services.) A change in physicians' fees results in a proportional change in the coinsurance amount, which affects the demand for physicians' services. The net effect of an increase in physicians' fees on the volume of services provided could be either positive or negative, depending on the relative magnitudes of the two supply-side effects (the substitution effect that increases work hours and the income effect that decreases work hours) and the demand-side coinsurance effect.[5]

Researchers have also proposed theories regarding volume responses in institutional settings, such as hospitals, nursing facilities, and laboratories. In those settings, volume responses have been characterized as firms' choosing their level of output in response to the payment rate, prices for medical inputs (primarily wages paid to their workers), and factors that affect demand. The key difference between firms' and physicians' choice of output level is that physicians have a demand for leisure time, whereas firms do not. Because of that difference, in the standard theoretical model of the behavior of an institutional provider, output would generally be assumed to rise in response to an increase in the payment rate and to fall in response to a decrease in the payment rate.[6]

One assumption underlying the analyses in this paper is that medical providers have some influence over the volume of medical services consumed. If that were not the case—if, for example, the consumption of medical services was determined solely by patients' preferences or by some objective assessment of medical "need"—then changes in payment rates would not be expected to affect the volume of services consumed. In fact, the availability of medical services has been shown to exert a strong influence over the volume of medical services consumed, in particular the volume of so-called supply-sensitive services.[7] In the specific case of post-acute care, the level of availability of different types of services has been shown to be a strong predictor of whether patients use post-acute care and what type of that care they use.[8]

Changes in Medicare's payment rates for SNF care could lead to supply-driven changes in the volume of SNF services provided. For example, in response to changes in Medicare's payment rates, SNFs could alter the availability of the care they provide through changes in the number of patients they treat, changes in their target mix of patients, or changes in their marketing practices (or all three). It is beyond the scope of this analysis to determine the exact mechanisms by which SNF volume could adjust in response to changes in payment rates, however.

Previous Empirical Research

Most of the recent empirical research on the volume response of health care providers has focused on the effect of fees paid to physicians on the volume of services provided by physicians.[9] The results of those studies are mixed: Some studies find that an increase in physicians' fees is associated with a decrease in the volume of services provided;[10] other studies find the opposite.[11]

Although hospitals account for a large share of total Medicare spending, there has been little empirical work done on volume responses in that setting. One recent paper found that increases in Medicare's payment rates for hospitals were associated with upcoding (toward diagnosis-related groups whose prices have been raised) rather than increases in the volume of admissions.[12] A separate study, which focused on the home health care setting, linked lower payment rates with a lower volume of home health care services.[13]

The lack of agreement in the empirical literature on physicians' volume response almost certainly stems, at least in part, from differences in research methods and data sources. That lack of agreement may also reflect the fact that the direction of the physicians' volume response is theoretically ambiguous and may, in reality, vary over time and across types of services. That theoretical ambiguity does not apply to services provided by institutions such as hospitals or nursing facilities. Perhaps as a consequence, the little research that has been done on those types of facilities points consistently toward volume varying positively with payment rates.

Medicare's Payment Rates for Skilled Nursing Facilities

From the 1980s through the mid-1990s, Medicare's outlays for SNFs increased rapidly. Between 1983 and 1997, annual growth in those outlays averaged 26 percent.[14] Since 1997, Medicare's system for paying for skilled nursing care has undergone a series of major revisions, with substantial impacts on the payment rates SNFs receive. Prior to those revisions, SNFs were paid by Medicare on a cost-reimbursement basis, meaning that SNFs were reimbursed for the actual costs they reported, subject to certain limits. Those limits were applied to routine costs, such as nursing and housekeeping, but not to ancillary services, such as physical and occupational therapy. As a result, Medicare's reimbursements to SNFs for ancillary services grew more rapidly than its reimbursements for routine costs.

In part to rein in Medicare's spending, lawmakers enacted the Balanced Budget Act of 1997, which replaced the cost-reimbursement system for SNFs with a prospective payment system. Under that system, SNFs are paid a fixed rate per resident per day.[15] The daily payment rate is set separately for different categories of residents and equals a national base rate multiplied by a local wage adjustor and a case-mix adjustor. The base rate is updated annually on the basis of changes in the SNF market basket (an index of input prices for SNFs calculated by the Centers for Medicare and Medicaid Services, or CMS). The local wage adjustor used by CMS in setting payment rates reflects differences across geographic regions in local hospital wages.[16] The case-mix adjustor is assigned separately to each SNF resident and reflects the estimated resource costs of caring for that resident.[17] To assign case-mix adjustors, CMS groups residents into resource utilization groups (RUGs) on the basis of a detailed assessment of each resident that is filled out by SNF staff.

After the initial implementation of the PPS, several large nursing facility chains reported large financial losses and filed for bankruptcy. In part, those bankruptcies prompted the Congress to pass an additional set of legislative changes that temporarily increased Medicare's SNF payment rates.[18] Both the Balanced Budget Refinement Act of 1999 (BBRA-1999) and the Benefits Improvement and Protection Act of 2000 (BIPA-2000) increased SNF payment rates across the board and also provided targeted increases for certain case-mix categories. For example, BBRA-1999 temporarily increased by 20 percent payment rates for 15 of the 44 RUGs. The expiration of those temporary increases in 2002 resulted in a decline in average payment rates between 2002 and 2003 (see Table 1).

The shift in Medicare's payment method for SNFs from cost reimbursement to prospective payment resulted in only fairly modest changes in the national average payment rates. The mean inflation-adjusted Medicare payment rate dropped from $357 in 1997 (pre-PPS) to $317 in 1999 (immediately post-PPS) and then rose again to $343 in 2001 (see Table 1). The impact on individual SNFs was much more varied; many experienced substantial increases in payment rates, but many others experienced sizable decreases.

In general, the introduction of the PPS compressed payment rates. That compression in the distribution of payment rates reflects the switch from a system in which payment rates depended on each SNF's costs to a system in which a uniform national formula was used (albeit with geographic-level and patient-level adjustors). SNFs that in the pre-PPS period had higher costs per patient-day (and, therefore, higher payment rates) generally faced declines in payment rates, whereas SNFs that had lower costs (and, therefore, lower payment rates) generally faced increases in payment rates.

Before the PPS was implemented, hospital-based SNFs received much higher payment rates, on average, than freestanding SNFs did. With the implementation of the PPS, therefore, they tended to face decreases in payment rates. Conversely, most freestanding SNFs faced increases in payment rates. Among both hospital-based and freestanding SNFs, however, there was a great deal of variation from one SNF to the next in the impact of the new system on payment rates.[19] The variation across SNFs both in the initial impact of the prospective payment system and in the impact of the changes from BBRA-1999 and BIPA-2000 provides a valuable opportunity for research into how SNFs respond to changes in payment rates.

Table 1. Medicare's Payment Rates for SNFs and the Volume of SNF Services Provided

	Geographic-Level Analysis		Provider-Level Analysis				
	1997	2001	1999	2000	2001	2002	2003
	Average Medicare Payment Rate (2003 dollars)						
All SNFs	357	343	317	316	343	348	315
Freestanding SNFs	332	341	308	311	341	350	317
Hospital-Based SNFs	463	350	356	344	350	338	303
Volume of SNF Services Provided (Days per beneficiary for geographic-level analysis and days per facility for provider-level analysis)							
All SNFs	1.36	1.35	2,786	2,933	3,275	3,649	3,964
Freestanding SNFs	1.11	1.18	2,659	2,846	3,215	3,636	3,983
Hospital-Based SNFs	0.25	0.17	3,550	3,506	3,700	3,741	3,806

Source: Congressional Budget Office analysis of Medicare administrative data.

Notes: SNF = skilled nursing facility.

Payment rates are inflated to the fourth quarter of 2003 using the national SNF market basket index. For the geographic-level analysis, payment rates and the volume of SNF services are calculated at the level of the hospital service area, and statistics are weighted by the number of fee-for-service beneficiaries in each area in 1997. For the provider-level analysis, payment rates and the volume of SNF services are calculated at the level of the SNF, and statistics are weighted by the average payments each SNF receives for Medicarecovered services. The number of SNFs included in the provider-level analysis is about 14,000 in each year.

METHODS FOR MEASURING THE VOLUME RESPONSE AMONG SKILLED NURSING FACILITIES

This paper uses two approaches to measure the effect on volume of changes in Medicare's SNF payment rates. The first is a geographic-level analysis, and the second is a provider-level analysis. Although those two empirical approaches are broadly similar, they use different data sets, units of analysis, and time periods. In both analyses, the percentage change in the volume of Medicare-covered SNF services is explained by the percentage change in the real (inflation-adjusted) payment rate and other control variables. Each approach identifies a component of the change in SNF payment rates that is directly attributable to changes in Medicare's payment formula and is not attributable to other factors (such as changes in the demographics of the SNF patient population or changes in the types of services provided by SNFs).

Both analyses focus exclusively on the services provided to Medicare beneficiaries who are enrolled in the traditional fee-for-service program. Medicare beneficiaries enrolled in private managed care plans (termed Medicare Advantage) are excluded because data on SNF volume and payment rates are not available for those beneficiaries. CBO chose to use resident-days, rather than spending or admissions, as the measure of the volume of SNF services because resident-days are used as Medicare's basis of payment for SNFs as well as Medicare beneficiaries' coinsurance payments for SNFs.

Empirical Specification for Both Analyses

The following general empirical specification is used in all the regression analyses in this paper:

$$\Delta Q_i = \beta \Delta P_i + X_i \gamma + \varepsilon_i$$

where i indexes either the geographic area or the SNF, ΔQ_i equals the arc percentage change in the volume of Medicare-covered SNF days, ΔP_i equals the arc percentage change in case-mix-constant real SNF payment rates, X_i includes a set of control variables, and ε_i is an error term. The change in SNF volume, ΔQ_i, is defined using an arc percentage change formula:

$$\Delta Q_i = \frac{Q_{i,t2} - Q_{i,t1}}{(Q_{i,t1} + Q_{i,t2})/2}$$

where the subscript $t1$ denotes the base year and $t2$ denotes a later year.[20]

The change in the SNF payment rate, ΔP_i, is also defined using an arc percentage change:

$$\Delta P_i = \frac{\sum_c P_{i,c,t2} Q_{i,c,t1} / I_{t2} - \sum_c P_{i,c,t1} Q_{i,c,t1} / I_{t1}}{\left(\sum_c P_{i,c,t2} Q_{i,c,t1} / I_{t2} + \sum_c P_{i,c,t1} Q_{i,c,t1} / I_{t1} \right)/2}$$

where the subscript c denotes a case-mix group (that is, a group of SNF residents with similar clinical characteristics and resource needs), where I_{t1} and I_{t2} denote a national index of input prices for SNFs, and where $P_{i,c,t}$ denotes the payment rate for unit i (either a geographic area or a SNF) for case-mix group c in time t.[21]

Defining the arc percentage change in SNF payment rates in that way holds the case mix constant using the base-year distribution and adjusts for inflation in prices of inputs. CBO's method for calculating the change in payment rates is referred to as a Laspeyres-type index because payment rates in the base year and the later year are both multiplied by the case-mix distribution in the base year. The change in the payment rate, ΔP_i, is attributable solely to real changes in payment rates within each case-mix group, rather than changes in the distribution of patients across case-mix groups.

In the regression analyses, the dependent variable, ΔQ_i, measures the arc percentage change in SNF volume. Because the dependent variable captures a change over time, the coefficient vector, γ, captures differential time trends that vary with the control variables included in X_i. The control variables in X_i include state indicator variables, an indicator for rural location, and an indicator for large urban location, as well as percentage changes in local real income per capita and local hospital wages.[22] The coefficients on the state indicator variables capture the impact of state-specific trends that might affect SNF utilization, such as changes in Medicaid's payment rates or changes in other health sectors, such as home health care.[23]

The coefficient of interest, β, captures the volume response, and it may be interpreted as follows. If, for example, β equals 0.2, then an increase of (arc) 1 percent in the payment rate (that is, ΔP_i equals 0.01) is associated with an increase of (arc) 0.2 percent in SNF volume (that is, the estimated ΔQ_i increases by 1 percent multiplied by 0.2).

In addition to estimating an overall SNF volume response, the analyses also estimate separate volume responses for hospital based and freestanding SNFs. In the geographic-level analysis, SNFs are first split into two groups, hospital based and freestanding, and then the changes in SNF volume and payment rates are calculated separately for those groups of SNFs, and separate regression models are run. In the provider-level analysis, separate regressions are run for hospital-based and freestanding SNFs. That approach allows the coefficient on the payment rate, β, and the vector of coefficients on the control variables, γ, to vary for hospital-based versus freestanding SNFs.

CBO used additional models to estimate separate volume responses for SNFs that received real increases and real decreases in payment rates. Two separate variables are used to capture the changes in payment rates: ΔP_i *increase*, which equals ΔP_i if the SNF or the geographic area faced an increase in the payment rate and equals zero, otherwise; and ΔP_i *decrease*, which equals ΔP_i if the SNF or the geographic area faced a decrease in the payment rate and zero, otherwise. The volume responses for increases and decreases in payment rates are calculated separately for hospital-based versus freestanding SNFs, which produces four separate volume response coefficients (increases to hospital-based SNFs, decreases to hospital-based SNFs, and so on).[24]

Specific Methods for the Geographic-Level Analysis

As a first step in the geographic-level analysis, CBO grouped Medicare fee-for-service beneficiaries into hospital service areas on the basis of their zip code of residence. HSAs, which were developed by the Center for the Evaluative Clinical Sciences at Dartmouth Medical School, represent local health care markets and are defined on the basis of observed patterns of health care utilization.[25] The analytical data set includes one observation for each HSA. There are 3,436 HSAs, and each has an average of around 10,000 Medicare fee-for-service beneficiaries.[26]

The volume of SNF services, which is measured at the HSA level in 1997 and 2001, equals the mean Medicare-covered SNF days per beneficiary per year. The volume of SNF services is defined on the basis of a beneficiary's residence; SNF days are attributed to the beneficiary's HSA regardless of the location of the SNF used. SNF volume is adjusted for beneficiaries' age and sex.[27] The year 1997 was chosen as the initial year because it was just before the prospective payment system was implemented; 2001 was chosen as the end year because the system had been phased in by then, and SNFs had had an opportunity to respond to the new payment rates.

For a given HSA, the arc percentage change in the payment rate is calculated on the basis of the payment rates for SNFs serving beneficiaries living in that HSA. To calculate that change in payment rates, case-mix-constant payment rates are first calculated for each SNF in 1997 and 2001, and then HSA-level payment rates are calculated as weighted means of the SNF-level payment rates. The first step is to calculate the mean SNF payment rate for each SNF in 1997. The second step is to simulate the mean payment rate for each SNF in 2001, assuming that each SNF's case mix is held constant.[28] Then HSA-level mean SNF payment rates are calculated for 1997 and 2001 from SNF-level payment rates using the following weight: the fraction of SNF days provided by each facility in 1997 to beneficiaries living in a given HSA. The HSA-level change in payment rates equals the arc percentage difference between the 1997 HSA-level mean payment rate and the simulated case-mix-constant 2001 payment rate. That arc percentage change is attributable solely to the implementation of the prospective payment system and does not reflect changes in SNFs' case mix or SNFs entering or exiting the market. For the geographic-level analysis, each HSA is weighted by the number of Medicare fee-for-service beneficiaries living in that HSA in 1997.

Data Sources for the Geographic-Level Analysis

Data on Medicare beneficiaries' zip code of residence, utilization of SNF services, and payments to SNFs are all taken from Medicare administrative records that include 100 percent of fee-for-service beneficiaries and SNF days. Beneficiaries' zip code of residence and fee-for-service enrollment are taken from the "Denominator" file, SNF utilization (Medicare-covered days and payments) is taken from the "MEDPAR" file, and SNF characteristics are taken from the "Provider of Services" file. County-level characteristics (urbanization and income) are taken from the 2004 Area Resource File (ARF).[29] The "crosswalk" from zip code to HSA is provided by the *Dartmouth Atlas of Health Care*.[30] Hospital wages are calculated from Medicare's hospital cost reports.

Specific Methods for the Provider-Level Analysis

The provider-level analysis measures the SNF volume response using data at the provider level from 1999 (the first full year after implementation of Medicare's new payment system) through 2003 (one year after the full transition to the PPS in 2002). The analysis reflects the payment add-ons by BBRA-1999 and BIPA-2000, which produced substantial price variations across SNFs (most of those add-ons ended in 2003).[31]

Table 2. Year-to-Year Changes in Total SNF Days from the Exit and Entry of SNFs, 1999 to 2003

	1999–2000	2000–2001	2001–2002	2002–2003
Total SNF Days (Millions)				
In originating year	41	43	48	53
In ending year	43	48	53	57
Change in total SNF days (Millions)	**1.9**	**4.7**	**5.1**	**4.5**
Days lost from exit of SNFs (Thousands)	435	386	388	444
Days gained from entry of SNFs (Thousands)	316	299	14	4
Net change in total SNF days (Thousands)	**-119**	**-87**	**-374**	**-440**
Net Change as a Percentage of				
Total SNF Days in Ending Year	-0.3	-0.2	-0.7	-0.8

Source: Congressional Budget Office analysis of Medicare administrative data.

Notes: SNF = skilled nursing facility.

A SNF is defined as an "entrant" if it provided Medicare-covered SNF services in a given year but not in the prior year, and it is defined as an "exiter" if it provided Medicare-covered SNF services in a given year but not in the next year.

Total SNF days are the number of Medicare-covered SNF days provided by all SNFs in a given year.

Volume is measured by the number of Medicare-covered SNF days provided by a given facility in a given year. The data set used for the provider-level analysis includes one observation for each combination of SNF and year-pair. For example, for a given SNF, there is one observation for 1999–2000 (changes in volume and payment rates are measured from 1999 to 2000), another observation for 2000–2001, and so forth. The changes in payment rates are calculated using a Laspeyres-type index, in which the mix of patients in the base year is used to generate an average payment rate in both the base year and the next year.

For SNFs that entered or exited the system during that five-year span, the arc percentage changes are calculated differently. A SNF is defined as an "entrant" if it provided Medicare-covered SNF services in a given year but not in the prior year, and it is defined as an "exiter" if it provided Medicare-covered SNF services in a given year but not in the next year. For exiters, the arc percentage changes in payment rate and volume are calculated using the standard formulas. For entrants, although it is possible to calculate the arc percentage change in volume using the standard formula, there is no information available on the distribution of patients across case-mix groups in the base year. Therefore, for entrants, the arc percentage change in payment rates in the year-pair in which they enter is calculated using a Paasche-type index, which incorporates the case-mix distribution in the later year.

The data show that the impact on total SNF days from the exit and entry of SNFs during the 1999–2003 period was not substantial (the net change was never larger than 1 percent; see Table 2). The net loss of days resulting from the exit of SNFs, however, increased throughout the period, rising from 0.3 percent of total days during the 1999–2000 period to 0.8 percent during the 2002–2003 period.

To examine whether SNFs responded differently to payment decreases than to payment increases, CBO created separate variables for increases and decreases in payment rates using the same approach as in the geographic-level analysis. In the provider-level analysis, each provider is weighted by payments it receives from Medicare-covered services.[32]

Data Sources for the Provider-Level Analysis

The primary data source for the provider-level analysis is a set of Medicare administrative records that summarize claims for each combination of SNF, case-mix group, and year. Payment rates are computed for each case-mix group within each facility for each year. Each facility's characteristics are taken from the "Provider of Services" file and Medicare's SNF cost reports. County-level characteristics (urbanization and income) are taken from the 2004 Area Resource File, and hospital wages are computed from Medicare's hospital cost reports.

RESULTS OF THE ANALYSES

The results of the geographic- and provider-level analyses indicate that the volume of SNF services varies positively with the SNF payment rate and that those responses occur among both freestanding and hospital-based SNFs. In both analyses, increases in payment rates are found to result in modest increases in volume. In the geographic-level analysis, decreases in payment rates are found to result in decreases in volume, whereas in the provider-level analysis, decreases in payment rates are found not to affect volume significantly.

Descriptive Statistics

CBO's analysis of Medicare administrative data provides descriptive statistics on the volume of SNF services and changes in SNF payment rates (all payment rates are expressed in 2003 dollars).

The geographic-level analysis shows that the mean Medicare payment per SNF day declined by 4 percent between 1997 and 2001, falling from $357 to $343, while the volume of SNF services was nearly unchanged at 1.36 days per beneficiary in 1997 and 1.35 days in 2001 (see the left panel of Table 1). In 1997, prior to the implementation of the prospective payment system, mean payment rates were much higher for hospital-based SNFs than for freestanding SNFs, $463 versus $332. By 2001, after the payment system had been fully implemented, that gap had almost entirely disappeared, reflecting a sharp drop in mean payment rates for hospital-based SNFs and a slight increase in mean payment rates for freestanding SNFs. The volume of hospital-based SNF services declined fairly sharply from 1997 to 2001, from 0.25 days per beneficiary to 0.17 days, while the volume of freestanding SNF services increased slightly, from 1.11 days to 1.18 days. It is notable that both payment rates and volume declined among hospital-based SNFs but increased among freestanding SNFs. That fact provides some preliminary evidence that SNF volume varies positively with the payment rate.

The provider-level analysis shows that in 2003, the mean SNF payment rate was almost identical to the mean payment rate in 1999 ($315 versus $317), but payment rates fluctuated sharply in the intervening years (see the right panel of Table 1). Changes legislated by BBRA-1999 and BIPA-2000 raised SNF payment rates in 2001 and 2002, but those rates dropped sharply in 2003. Mean SNF days for each facility increased substantially from 1999 to 2003, particularly among freestanding SNFs.

CBO's analysis also shows the distribution of the changes in Medicare's payment rates. In the geographic-level analysis, there is a great deal of variation in the distribution of changes in payment rates across areas—at the 90th percentile, the SNF payment rate increased by 23.2 percent, whereas at the 10th percentile, the SNF payment rate decreased by 33.0 percent (see Figure 1). In the provider-level analysis, the distribution of changes in payment rates is narrower, but there is still a substantial amount of variation across SNFs and from year-pair to year-pair (see Figure 2).

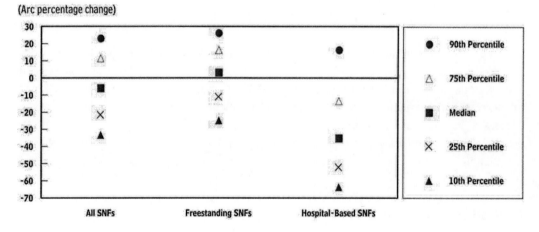

Figure 1. Changes in Medicare's Payment Rates, 1997 to 2001, Based on CBO's Geographic-Level Analysis

Source: Congressional Budget Office analysis of Medicare administrative data.
Notes: SNF = skilled nursing facility.

This figure presents statistics on the distribution of the arc percentage changes in Medicare's case-mix-constant payment rates for SNFs. All payment rates are inflated to the fourth quarter of 2003 using the national SNF market basket index. Changes in payment rates are calculated at the level of the hospital service area, and statistics are weighted by the number of fee-for-service beneficiaries in each area in 1997.

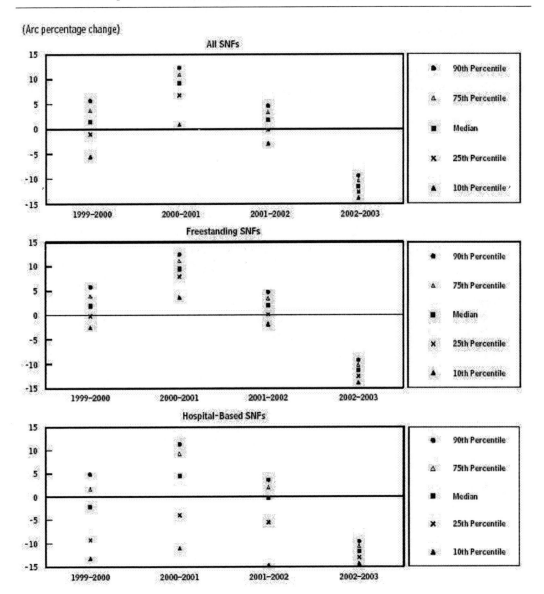

Figure 2. Year-to-Year Changes in Medicare's Payment Rates, 1999 to 2003, Based on CBO's Provider-Level Analysis

Source: Congressional Budget Office analysis of Medicare administrative data.
Notes: SNF = skilled nursing facility.

This figure presents statistics on the distribution of the arc percentage changes in Medicare's case-mix-constant payment rates for SNFs. All payment rates are inflated to the fourth quarter of 2003 using the national SNF market basket index. Changes in payment rates are calculated at the level of the SNF, and statistics are weighted by the average payments each SNF receives for Medicarecovered services. The number of SNFs included in this analysis is about 14,000 in each year.

Key Results for the Geographic-Level Analysis

The key regression results for the geographic-level analysis indicate that increases in SNF payment rates are associated with a statistically significant increase in SNF volume and that decreases in payment rates are associated with decreases in volume (see the left panel of Table 3). Among all SNFs, a change of 1 percent in the SNF payment rate is associated with a change in SNF volume of 0.13 percent. Compared with the volume-response coefficient for freestanding SNFs, the coefficient for hospital-based SNFs is found to be larger (0.26), which implies that hospital-based SNFs are more responsive than freestanding SNFs to changes in payment rates. Among hospital-based SNFs, both those facing increases in payment rates and those facing decreases in payment rates exhibited similar responses, with volume in both cases changing in the same direction as the change in the payment rate.[33] Among freestanding SNFs, the coefficients on increases and decreases in payment rates are not individually statistically significant, but they are jointly statistically significant, and both point estimates are similar to the overall volume response.

Table 3. Estimated Volume Responses Among SNFs to Changes of 1 Percent in Medicare's Payment Rates

(Percent)	Geographic-Level Analysis	Provider-Level Analysis
All SNFs	0.13 ***	0.23 ***
Freestanding	0.08 **	0.22 ***
Hospital-based	0.26 ***	0.08
Freestanding SNFs		
Increase in payment rate	0.06	0.30 ***
Decrease in payment rate	0.10	0.10
Hospital-based SNFs		
Increase in payment rate	0.43 ***	0.39 ***
Decrease in payment rate	0.20 ***	-0.06

Source: Congressional Budget Office analysis of Medicare administrative data.
Notes: SNF = skilled nursing facility; ** = p-value < 0.05; *** = p-value < 0.01.
   This table presents the key coefficients for a set of regression models. In each regression model, the dependent variable is the arc percentage change in the volume of Medicare-covered SNF services. In the geographic-level analysis, the volume of SNF services is measured by the number of Medicare-covered SNF days per beneficiary. In the provider-level analysis, the volume of SNF services is measured by the number of Medicare-covered SNF days provided by each facility. The statistics presented in this table are the coefficients on the arc percentage change in Medicare's real payment rate for SNFs. A higher volumeresponse coefficient implies a more responsive SNF. For the geographic-level analysis, beneficiaries are grouped into hospital service areas on the basis of their zip code of residence, and regressions are weighted by the number of fee-for-service beneficiaries in each area in 1997. For the provider-level analysis, regressions are weighted by the average payments each SNF receives for Medicare-covered services.

Key Results for the Provider-Level Analysis

The results of the provider-level analysis provide further evidence of the existence of a statistically significant volume response (see the right panel of Table 3). In the analysis including all SNFs, the coefficient on the change in the payment rate is 0.23, which implies that a change of 1 percent in the SNF payment rate would lead to a change in volume of 0.23 percent in the same direction as the change in the payment rate. In the provider-level analysis, the volume response is found to be statistically significant only among freestanding SNFs. When increases and decreases in payment rates are analyzed separately, increases in payment rates are found to result in increases in volume among both freestanding and hospital-based SNFs, but decreases in payment rates are not associated with statistically significant changes in volume

DISCUSSION OF THE RESULTS

Both the geographic-level analysis and the provider-level analysis indicate that the volume of Medicare-covered SNF services varies positively with the payment rate, that the magnitude of the response is fairly modest, and that the response occurs both among freestanding and hospital-based SNFs. Although the provider-level analysis suggests that SNF volume responds only to increases in payment rates, the geographic-level analysis suggests that SNFs respond, in a roughly symmetrical fashion, to both increases and decreases in payment rates.

One possible explanation for that finding is that increases in volume in response to higher payment rates might occur over a relatively short time frame, whereas decreases in volume in response to lower payment rates might occur over a longer time frame. The geographic-level analysis is suited to detecting long-run responses to changes in payment rates (because it measures the four-year response from 1997 to 2001), whereas the provider-level analysis is better suited to detecting short-run responses (because it measures annual responses from 1999 to 2003).

The difference between the overall volume response estimated in the geographic-level analysis (0.13) and the response estimated in the provider-level analysis (0.23) is not statistically significant, although it deserves some comment. The difference between those two estimates could reflect different time periods,[34] different levels of measurement error in the two types of analyses, or a bias in one or both of the analyses.[35]

The difference in estimated volume responses could also reflect a certain type of volume spillover effect. Suppose that there are two SNFs in the same geographic area and that one SNF receives a payment increase and the other does not. Based on the provider-level analysis, the SNF that receives the increase in payment rate is predicted to increase its volume relative to the SNF that receives no change in payment rate. One possible spillover effect of one SNF taking steps to increase its volume could be to draw some volume away from other SNFs in the same area. The change in volume as measured in the geographic-level analysis would reflect the combination of both the main effect (an increase in volume at the SNF that received a payment increase) and the volume spillover effect (a decrease in volume at the SNF that received no change in payment rate). That type of spillover effect could explain the finding of a larger volume response in the provider-level analysis than in the geographic-level analysis.

The results of this research indicate that the volume of SNF services varies positively with changes in Medicare's payment rate. However, the total effect on Medicare's SNF spending of a change in Medicare's payment rate would also include the impact on the "intensity" of services. Intensity, as it is generally defined, is a measure of the average complexity and costliness of medical services. In the SNF setting, changes in intensity would result from changes over time in the shares of residents assigned to different case-mix categories. (Each case-mix category is assigned a separate payment rate.)

One potential topic for future research is the possible existence of spillover effects from changes in payment rates for SNFs on the volume of services provided in other types of health care facilities. Other topics of interest include volume responses in institutional settings besides SNFs, such as hospitals and home health agencies. Volume responses, particularly in the hospital setting, are directly relevant to projections of the impact on Medicare's spending of changes in payment rates.

APPENDIX: DETAILED REGRESSION RESULTS

This appendix presents detailed regression results (see Tables A-1 and A-2) from the Congressional Budget Office's geographic-level analysis and provider-level analysis of how the volume of Medicare-covered skilled nursing facility (SNF) services adjusts in response to changes in Medicare's SNF payment rates. In both sets of analyses, the dependent variable is the arc percentage change in the volume of Medicare-covered SNF days, and the key independent variable is the case-mix-constant arc percentage change in Medicare's real (inflation-adjusted) payment rate for SNFs. For the geographic-level analysis, the unit of the analysis is the hospital service area ($N = 3,436$), and changes in volume and payment rates are measured from 1997 to 2001. For the provider-level analysis, the unit of analysis is the SNF, and changes in volume and payment rates are measured for each year-pair from 1999 through 2003 (1999–2000, 2000–2001, and so on).

Table A.1. Detailed Regression Results from CBO's Geographic-Level Analysis

Variable	SNF Days per Beneficiary for All SNFs	SNF Days per Beneficiary for Freestanding SNFs		SNF Days per Beneficiary for Hospital Based SNFs	
		First Regression	Second Regression	First Regression	Second Regression
Arc Percentage Change in Medicare's Payment Rate for SNFs[a]	0.130*** (0.029)				
Arc percentage change in Medicare's payment rate for freestanding SNFs		0.079** (0.036)			
Arc percentage change in Medicare's payment rate for freestanding SNFs x "increase" indicator[b]			0.065 (0.052)		
Arc percentage change in Medicare's payment rate for freestanding SNFs x "decrease" indicator[b]			0.098 (0.062)		
Arc percentage change in Medicare's payment rate for hospital-based SNFs				0.256*** (0.040)	
Arc percentage change in					0.429*** (0.107)
Medicare's payment rate for hospital-based SNFs x "increase" indicator[b]					

Table A.1. (Continued)

Variable	SNF Days per Beneficiary for All SNFs	SNF Days per Beneficiary for Freestanding SNFs		SNF Days per Beneficiary for Hospital Based SNFs	
		First Regression	Second Regression	First Regression	Second Regression
Arc percentage change in Medicare's payment rate for hospital-based SNFs x "decrease" indicator[b]					0.197*** (0.053)
Rural Indicator[c]	0.020* (0.011)	0.015 (0.013)	0.015 (0.013)	0.080*** (0.027)	0.074*** (0.027)
Large Urban Indicator[c]	-0.023** (0.009)	-0.003 (0.011)	-0.003 (0.011)	-0.052** (0.024)	-0.053** (0.024)
Arc Percentage Change from 1997 to 2001 in Hospital Wages[d]	-0.032 (0.046)	-0.038 (0.055)	-0.038 (0.055)	0.028 (0.120)	0.035 (0.120)
Arc Percentage Change from 1997 to 2001 in Real (CPI-inflated) Income per Capita[e]	-0.322*** (0.074)	-0.371*** (0.089)	-0.372*** (0.089)	0.015 (0.194)	0.005 (0.194)
Estimated Difference Between Coefficients on "Increases" and "Decreases"			-0.033 (0.088)		0.232* (0.133)
F-statistic on Exclusion of Both "Increases" and "Decreases" in Payment Rates			4.99**		36.24***
Number of Observations	3,435	3,424	3,424	3,396	3,396
R-squared	0.326	0.244	0.244	0.250	0.251

Source: Congressional Budget Office analysis of Medicare administrative data.

Notes: SNF = skilled nursing facility; * = p-value < 0.10; ** = p-value < 0.05; *** = p- value < 0.01; CPI = the consumer price index for all urban consumers.

Standard errors are shown in parentheses. All regressions are weighted by the number of fee-for-service beneficiaries in each hospital service area (HSA) in 1997. State indicator variables are included in each regression (coefficient estimates are not shown).

a. All payment rates are inflated to the fourth quarter of 2003 using the national SNF market basket index.

b. For each HSA, an "increase" indicator and a "decrease" indicator are defined separately for freestanding and hospital-based SNFs depending on whether the arc percentage change in Medicare's input price-inflated payment rate for that type of SNF is positive or negative. The sign of the reported coefficients, however, reflects the effect of an increase in the payment rate.

c. The "small urban" reference category is omitted.

d. Hospital wages are measured by aggregating salaries and hours for all hospitals in each HSA. For HSAs that do not contain a hospital, hospital wages are measured by aggregating all hospitals in the hospital referral region in which the HSA is located. Hospital referral regions are aggregations of HSAs that represent regional health care markets.

e. County-level income per capita is measured using the 2004 Area Resource File. The county-level income measures are aggregated to the HSA level using as weights the fraction of all Medicare beneficiaries living in each HSA who lived in the county in 1997.

Table A.2. Detailed Regression Results from CBO's Provider-Level Analysis

Variable	SNF Days per Facility for All SNFs	SNF Days per Facility for Freestanding SNFs		SNF Days per Facility for Hospital-Based SNFs	
		First Regression	Second Regression	First Regression	Second Regression
Arc Percentage Change in Medicare's Payment Rate[a]	0.227*** (0.030)	0.219*** (0.040)		0.079 (0.052)	
Arc percentage change in Medicare's payment rate x "increase" indicator[b]			0.302*** (0.060)		0.392*** (0.132)
Arc percentage change in Medicare's payment rate x "decrease" indicator[b]			0.104 (0.073)		-0.058 (0.074)
Rural Indicator[c]	0 (0.004)	-0.004 (0.004)	-0.004 (0.004)	0.015 (0.009)	0.013 (0.009)
Large Urban Indicator[c]	0.003 (0.003)	0.005* (0.003)	0.005* (0.003)	-0.012 (0.008)	-0.012 (0.008)
Arc Percentage Change from 1997 to 2001 in Hospital Wages[d]	0.021 (0.018)	0.031 (0.020)	0.031 (0.020)	-0.035 (0.053)	-0.033 (0.053)
Arc Percentage Change from 1997 to 2001 in Real (CPI-inflated) Income per Capita[e]	-0.182*** (0.055)	-0.105* (0.060)	-0.105* (0.060)	-0.568*** (0.149)	-0.559*** (0.149)
Year-Pair Indicator					
1999-2000[f]	-0.048*** (0.005)	-0.044*** (0.006)	-0.033*** (0.009)	-0.037*** (0.010)	-0.031*** (0.010)
2000-2001[f]	-0.002 (0.007)	-0.004 (0.009)	0.001 (0.009)	0.050*** (0.012)	0.046*** (0.012)
2001-2002[f]	0.002 (0.005)	0.006 (0.006)	0.017** (0.008)	0 (0.010)	0.007 (0.011)
Hospital-Based Indicator[g]	-0.104*** (0.004)				
Nonprofit Indicator[h]	-0.003 (0.006)	0.015* (0.008)	0.015* (0.008)	-0.019** (0.010)	-0.018* (0.010)

Table A.2. (Continued)

Variable	SNF Days per Facility for All SNFs	SNF Days per Facility for Freestanding SNFs		SNF Days per Facility for Hospital-Based SNFs	
		First Regression	Second Regression	First Regression	Second Regression
For-Profit Indicator[h]	-0.006 (0.006)	0.007 (0.008)	0.007 (0.008)	-0.008 (0.013)	-0.008 (0.013)
Estimated Difference Between Coefficient on "Increases" and "Decreases"			0.198* (0.105)		0.451*** (0.175)
F-statistic on Exclusion of Changes in Payment Rates for "Increases" and "Decreases"			24.16***		7.27***
Number of Observations	52,265	46,016	46,016	6,249	6,249
R-squared	0.050	0.036	0.036	0.049	0.050

Source: Congressional Budget Office analysis of Medicare administrative data.

Notes: SNF = skilled nursing facility; * = p-value < 0.10; ** = p-value < 0.05; *** = p-value < 0.01; CPI = the consumer price index for all urban consumers.

Standard errors are shown in parentheses. All regressions are weighted by each SNF's average Medicare expenditures. State indicator variables and indicator variables for the top 10 national chains are included in each regression (coefficient estimates are not shown).

a. All payment rates are inflated to the fourth quarter of 2003 using the national SNF market basket index.

b. Each SNF is defined as receiving an "increase" or a "decrease" separately for each year-pair depending on whether the arc percentage change in Medicare's input price-inflated payment rate for that SNF is positive or negative. The sign of the reported coefficients, however, reflects the effect of an increase in the payment rate.

c. The "small urban" reference category is omitted.

d. Hospital wages are measured by aggregating salaries and hours for all hospitals in each county. For counties that do not contain a hospital, corresponding state average hospital wages are used.

e. County-level income per capita is measured using the 2004 Area Resource File.

f. The "2002–2003 year-pair" reference category is omitted.

g. The "freestanding" reference category is omitted.

h. The "government-owned" reference category is omitted.

End Notes

[1] Congressional Budget Office, "Fact Sheet for CBO's March 2007 Baseline: Medicare (Components of Benefits Payments)," p. 2.

[2] Medicare Payment Advisory Commission, *Report to Congress: Medicare Payment Policy* (March 2007), p. 171.

[3] In cases in which a decrease in the payment rate has been found to lead to an increase in volume, the volume response has been referred to in the literature as a "volume offset." That term is used because some of the savings to Medicare from the decrease in payment rates would be offset by the increase in volume.

[4] See, for example, Thomas G. McGuire and Mark V. Pauly, "Physician Response to Fee Changes with Multiple Payers," *Journal of Health Economics*, vol. 10, no. 4 (1991), pp. 385–410.

[5] Congressional Budget Office, Factors *Underlying the Growth in Medicare's Spending for Physicians' Services* (June 2007).

[6] For a theoretical analysis of hospitals' responses to payment changes and a summary of early evidence on the effects of Medicare's PPS for hospitals, see Dominic Hodgkin and Thomas G. McGuire, "Payment Levels and Hospital Response to Prospective Payment," *Journal of Health Economics*, vol. 13, no. 1 (March 1994), pp. 1–29. A volume offset could occur in the hospital setting if a hospital, facing a reduction in the payment rate, increased its output to maintain its total revenues. That type of behavior might be expected if the hospital had large fixed costs and was concerned primarily with its own survival rather than maximizing its profits.

[7] John E. Wennberg, Elliott S. Fisher, and Jonathan S. Skinner, "Geography and the Debate over Medicare Reform," *Health Affairs*, Web exclusive (February 13, 2002), pp. W96–W114.

[8] Melinda Beeuwkes Buntin and others, *How Much Is Post-Acute Care Use Affected by Its Availability?* Working Paper No. 10424 (Cambridge, Mass.: National Bureau of Economic Research, 2004), available at http://papers.nber.org/papers/w10424.pdf.

[9] Several decades ago, prior to the rise of managed care and government-run administered pricing systems, physicians had a great deal of discretion over the fees they charged and the payment rates they received. In that context, an appropriate model of physicians' volume responses would treat both the volume of physicians' services and payment rates as jointly determined outcomes of interest (see, for example, Martin S. Feldstein, "The Rising Price of Physicians' Services," *Review of Economics and Statistics*, vol. 52, no. 2, May 1970, pp. 121–133; and Mark V. Pauly and Mark A. Satterthwaite, "The Pricing of Primary Care Physicians Services: A Test of the Role of Consumer Information," *Bell Journal of Economics*, vol. 12, no. 2, Autumn 1981, pp. 488–506). More-recent research on physicians' volume responses, reflecting the institutional changes that have occurred, generally assumes that payment rates are not chosen by the physician or patients and that physicians and patients respond to externally driven changes in payment rates.

[10] Sandra Christensen, "Volume Responses to Exogenous Changes in Medicare's Payment Policies," *Health Services Research*, vol. 27, no. 1 (April 1992), pp. 65–79; Xuan Nguyen Nguyen and Frederick William Derrick, "Physician Behavioral Response to a Medicare Price Reduction," *Health Services Research*, vol. 32, no. 3 (August 1997), pp. 283–298; and Winnie C. Yip, "Physician Response to Medicare Fee Reductions: Changes in the Volume of Coronary Artery Bypass Graft (CABG) Surgeries in the Medicare and Private Sectors," *Journal of Health Economics*, vol. 17, no. 6 (December 1998), pp. 675–699.

[11] Jon Gruber and others, "Physician Fees and Procedure Intensity: The Case of Cesarean Delivery," *Journal of Health Economics*, vol. 18, no. 4 (August 1999), pp. 473–490; Jean M. Mitchell and others, "Spillover Effects of Medicare Fee Reductions: Evidence from Ophthalmology," *International Journal of Health Care Finance and Economics*, vol. 2, no. 3 (2002), pp. 171–188; and Jean M. Mitchell and others, "Physicians' Responses to Medicare Fee Schedule Reductions," *Medical Care*, vol. 38, no. 10 (2000), pp. 1029–1039.

[12] Leemore S. Dafny, "How Do Hospitals Respond to Price Changes?" *American Economic Review*, vol. 95, no. 5 (December 2005), pp. 1525–1547.

[13] Robin McKnight, *Home Care Reimbursement, Long-Term Care Utilization, and Health Outcomes*, Working Paper No. 10414 (Cambridge, Mass.: National Bureau of Economic Research, 2004), available at http://papers.nber.org/papers/w10414.pdf.

[14] Centers for Medicare and Medicaid Services, "2006 Medicare and Medicaid Statistical Supplement," available at www.cms.hhs.gov/ MedicareMedicaidStatSupp/.

[15] Each SNF began the transition to the new payment system beginning with its first cost-reporting period on or after July 1, 1998. During the three-year transition period, part of the payment rate that each SNF received was based on the facility's specific historical unit cost. By fiscal year 2002, all SNFs were paid the PPS federal rate.

[16] CBO includes in the regression analyses a measure of the change over time in local hospital wages (measured by aggregating salaries and hours for all hospitals in each county or HSA). That measure differs from the wage adjustor used by CMS in setting payment rates. CBO calculated changes over time in the wages paid by hospitals during the periods corresponding to the changes in SNF volume. The local wage adjustor calculated by CMS was not used because, by the time it could have been applied in setting payment rates, it would have been based on data that were several years out of date.

[17] Julie Stone, *Medicare's Skilled Nursing Facility Payment*, CRS Report for Congress RL33921 (March 14, 2007), available at www.congress.gov/erp/rl/pdf/RL33921.pdf. At different times during a single stay, SNF residents may be assigned to different case-mix categories if their resident assessments change over the course of their stay.

[18] For a discussion of the bankruptcies and the adequacy of Medicare's payment rates for SNFs, see the statement of Laura A. Dummit, Associate Director, Health Financing and Public Health Issues, Health, Education, and Human Services Division, General Accounting Office (now the Government Accountability Office), before the Senate Special Committee on Aging, *Nursing Homes: Aggregate Medicare Payments Are Adequate Despite Bankruptcies*, GAO/T-HEHS-00-192 (September 5, 2000), available at www.gao.gov/archive/2000/he00192t.pdf.

[19] The average SNF payment rate (in 2003 dollars and keeping the case mix constant) declined by 4.7 percent during the 1997–2001 period but by only 2.1 percent during the 1999–2003 period. One measure of variation—the range in payment rate changes between the 75th and 25th percentiles—was 44.6 percent in the former period and 20.4 percent during the latter period. (Those data underlie Figures 1 and 2.)

[20] Arc percentage changes are used rather than simple percentage changes $((Q_{i,t2} - Q_{i,t1})/Q_{i,t1})$ or natural logarithm-based changes $(l_n(Q_{i,t2}/Q_{i,t1})$ for two reasons: First, the arc percentage change,1 is defined (that is, nonmissing) even when volume is zero in either the base year or the later year; and, second, the arc percentage change is naturally bounded by the range [-2, 2], which reduces the need to screen for extreme values.

[21] All payment rates are inflated to the fourth quarter of 2003 using the national SNF market basket index.

[22] Income per capita is inflated using the consumer price index for all urban consumers. The percentage change in hospital wages is used as a proxy for local changes in SNFs' input prices. The provider-level analysis includes additional controls that are not in the geographic-level analysis: an indicator variable for whether the SNF is hospital based, an indicator variable for nonprofit ownership, an indicator variable for for-profit ownership (the government-owned reference category is omitted), and an indicator variable for whether the SNF is a member of a large national chain (independence from a large chain is the reference category).

[23] Several major changes to Medicare policy were implemented around the same time as the new prospective payment system for SNFs. Those changes include clarification of the eligibility standards for Medicare's home health benefit and transitions to prospective payment for the following types of providers: home health agencies, hospital outpatient departments, inpatient rehabilitation facilities, long-term care hospitals, and psychiatric facilities. The impact of the changes in the home health care sector was particularly striking, with Medicare's spending on home health care falling by more than half from 1997 to 1999 and then rebounding sharply beginning in 2001. The changes occurring in sectors outside SNFs may have affected trends in SNF utilization if SNFs have the potential to serve as substitutes for those other sectors. The state indicator variables are included in the analyses to help control for the changes that were occurring in other sectors.

[24] In the geographic-level analysis, areas with large concentrations of hospital-based SNFs are highly correlated with areas facing a payment rate decrease. Estimating responses to increases and decreases separately for hospital-based versus freestanding SNFs helps avoid confusing the effect of having a large concentration of hospital-based SNFs with the effect of facing a decrease in payment rates. In the provider-level analysis, however, because hospital-based SNFs are more likely than freestanding SNFs to experience decreases in payment rates, controlling for hospital-based and freestanding SNFs can be done directly by including the hospital-based/freestanding fixed effects and their interactions with the price variable on the right-hand side of the regression equation.

[25] Dartmouth Medical School, Center for the Evaluative Clinical Sciences, *The Dartmouth Atlas of Health Care* (Hanover, N.H.: American Hospital Publishing, 1996).

[26] In 2002, 90 percent of HSAs had a Medicare fee-for-service population of between 700 and 37,000.

[27] To adjust SNF volume for beneficiaries' demographics, the volume of SNF services (SNF days per beneficiary) is first measured for the year 1998 for different demographic cells. Those demographic cells are defined by combinations of age group (under 65, 65 to 74, 75 to 84, and 85 and up) and sex. The 1998 SNF volume by demographic cell is then multiplied by the number of beneficiaries in each HSA in each demographic cell in each year— that calculation yields a predicted SNF volume for each HSA for each year. The adjusted SNF volume for a given HSA is then calculated by multiplying the actual SNF volume in the HSA by the inverse of the ratio of predicted SNF volume in that HSA to the national mean SNF volume for that year.

[28] Simulated 2001 payment rates are used instead of observed 2001 payment rates, for several reasons. A mean payment rate could be calculated for each SNF for 2001, but the differences between the observed 1997 payment rates and the observed 2001 payment rates reflect not just legislative changes to Medicare's payment formula (which is the focus of the analysis) but also changes in SNFs' patient populations and in the services SNFs provide. In addition, some SNFs exited the market between 1997 and 2001; for those facilities, the mean 2001 payment rate cannot be calculated. A detailed explanation of the process of simulating 2001 payment rates for each SNF is available in Chapin White, "Medicare's New Prospective Payment System for Skilled Nursing Facilities: Effects on Staffing and Quality of Care," *Inquiry*, vol. 43, no. 1 (Winter 2005/2006), pp. 351–366.

[29] The county-level data from the ARF are aggregated to generate HSA-level measures by taking the weighted means of the county-level measures (using as the weight the fraction of Medicare fee-for-service beneficiaries living in a given HSA who also live in a given county).

[30] Dartmouth Medical School, Center for the Evaluative Clinical Sciences, *Zip Code to HSA to HRR Crosswalk File* (accessed May 15, 2003).

[31] The real average payment per day declined by 9.5 percent in 2003 (see Table 1). That drop would have been even larger had RUG refinement been implemented in 2003. (The 20 percent increase to 15 RUG groups and the 6.7 percent increase to 14 rehabilitation RUG groups initiated by BBRA-1999 and BIPA-2000 still remained in 2003 because RUG refinement was not implemented that year.)

[32] Several edits are performed on the provider-level data to limit the influence of observations with extreme values. First, an editing screen is used to identify and remove observations with unusual changes in volume or payment rate. Second, observations that are found to be very highly influential in the basic model are removed from all provider-level analyses. Those edits are based on information in David A. Belsley and others, *Regression Diagnostics: Identifying Influential Data and Sources of Collinearity* (New York: Wiley-Interscience, 1980).

[33] Among hospital-based SNFs, the magnitude of the volume response is larger among SNFs facing increases in payment rates than among those facing decreases (0.43 versus 0.20), but the difference is only weakly statistically significant (the p-value is less than 0.10).

[34] By examining the 1997–2001 period, the geographic-level analysis largely estimated the response of SNFs to Medicare's transition from a cost-based system to a prospective payment system. In contrast, the provider-level analysis, by focusing on the 1999–2003 period, estimated the response of SNFs to Medicare's payment changes under the PPS.

[35] Measurement error in an independent variable will result in a bias toward zero in the estimated coefficient on that variable in a regression analysis. The discrepancy between the estimated volume responses could be explained by the greater degree of error in the measurement of changes in payment rates in the geographic-level analysis versus the provider-level analysis.

In: Medicare: A Primer
Editor: Alice R. Williamson

ISBN: 978-1-60741-108-6
© 2009 Nova Science Publishers, Inc.

Chapter 2

FACTORS UNDERLYING THE GROWTH IN MEDICARE'S SPENDING FOR PHYSICIAN'S SERVICES

United States Congressional Budget Office

SUMMARY AND INTRODUCTION

The central long-term fiscal challenge facing the nation involves rising costs in Medicare, Medicaid, and other federal health-related programs. The Congressional Budget Office (CBO) is therefore expanding its work in examining the rising costs within the nation's federal health programs as well as possible policy responses. One rapidly growing component of Medicare involves payments for physicians' services, which is the focus of this paper.

Medicare compensates physicians for services they provide under the Supplemental Medical Insurance program, or Medicare Part B, on the basis of a fee schedule that specifies payment rates for each type of covered service. Payment rates are calculated in three steps: First, the fee schedule stipulates relative value units (RVUs), which measure the resources required to provide a given service. Second, payments are adjusted to account for geographical differences in input prices. Third, a "conversion factor" translates the geographically adjusted RVUs for a particular service into a dollar amount.

Annual updates to payment rates are governed by a mechanism known as the Sustainable Growth Rate (SGR), which aims to control Medicare's outlays for physicians' services.[1] Established in the Balanced Budget Act of 1997 (Public Law 105-33) and implemented in 1998, the SGR formula operates by setting a target amount for such expenditures and adjusting payment rates to reflect differences between actual spending and spending targets (both of which are measured on an annual and a cumulative basis). If actual spending under the SGR does not deviate from the expenditure targets, payment rates under the physician fee schedule are simply increased by the percentage change in the Medicare economic index, or MEI.[2] However, if actual spending is above the targets set by the SGR formula, the update to payment rates will be smaller than the increase in the MEI. If spending is below the targets, the update will be higher than the increase in the MEI. Those adjustments are designed so that, over a period of several years, cumulative spending will be brought into line with the cumulative expenditure target.

Annual updates to payment rates for physicians' services have varied widely in recent years, ranging from a minimum of about -5 percent (in 1999 and in 2002) to a maximum of roughly 5 percent (in 2000). (When adjusted to account for changes in the MEI, updates to payment rates have ranged from about -8 percent to 3 percent.) According to CBO's estimates, if provisions of current law remained unchanged, Medicare's payments to physicians would be reduced by about 10 percent in 2008 and by about 5 percent annually over the following several years. However, because lawmakers overrode the SGR mechanism between 2003 and 2007—replacing negative updates with small positive or zero updates—it is uncertain whether the SGR mechanism will be allowed to operate as specified.

Although updates to Medicare's payment rates have fluctuated since the SGR was established, spending for physicians' services under the fee schedule has increased steadily, rising by 79.2 percent between 1997 and 2005. Even after adjusting for changes in the cost of providing physicians' services—as measured by the Medicare economic index—and for growth in the number of beneficiaries enrolled in the program, spending on physicians' services has increased by 34.5 percent.[3]

Evaluating Changes in Program Spending

In this background paper, CBO examines Medicare's payments to physicians over the period in which the SGR mechanism has been in place, in order to better understand and project future changes in program spending. The analysis focuses on three issues:

- First, it breaks down annual changes in spending into two components: those attributable to changes in the rates that Medicare pays physicians for their services and those attributable to changes in the volume and intensity of services provided.[4] It then examines the relative importance of each component in explaining overall program growth.

- Second, it focuses on changes in the components of Medicare's payments rates for physicians' services, in order to assess the impact of such changes on spending growth over time.

- Third, the paper estimates the secular trend in the volume and intensity of services provided by physicians and considers the analytical issue of how physicians and beneficiaries respond to changes in Medicare's payment rates. Specifically, the analysis evaluates the portion of observed increases in the quantity of services provided to Medicare beneficiaries that is attributable to an underlying trend and the portion that is attributable to behavioral responses on the part of physicians and beneficiaries. (A behavioral response to a change in Medicare's payment rates might occur, for example, if physicians responded to a reduction in those rates by increasing the volume or intensity of their services in order to offset a potential decline in income; the opposite might occur if payment rates were increased. A behavioral response might also occur if changes in physicians' payment rates, which result in changes in beneficiaries' copayments, caused those beneficiaries to increase or decrease the amounts of services they required.)

This paper differs from previous research in a number of ways: It covers a greater number of years with persistent changes in payment rates (both positive and negative), which affected all physicians (and beneficiaries) who participated in the program. In addition, CBO's analysis was conducted at the aggregate level rather than at the individual physician or practice level; thus, it is more directly applicable to budgetary analysis.

Interpreting the Results

The analysis finds that, between 1997 and 2005, the 34.5 percent observed growth in Medicare's per-beneficiary spending, as adjusted by the Medicare economic index, is explained by growth in the volume and intensity of physicians' services rather than by changes in Medicare's payment rates. In fact, the quantity of services that physicians provided during that period increased by slightly more (39.4 percent) than did Medicare's per-beneficiary spending on physicians' services. Conversely, after medical price inflation, as measured by the MEI, is taken into account, Medicare's payment rates for such services actually declined slightly during that period.

The decline in Medicare's payment rates during that period is attributable to SGR-related changes in the conversion factor. Those changes offset other factors in Medicare's pricing system that would have led to higher payment rates. In terms of the quantity of services provided by physicians, CBO finds an annual trend of approximately 4 percent and a behavioral response that offsets 28 percent of the potential revenue change due to changes in payment rates. For example, if changes in payment rates alone—independent of the effects of a behavioral response—were to cause physicians' revenues to decline by $1,000 per year, the analysis is consistent with physicians' recouping about $280 of that projected loss by increasing the volume or intensity of their services. An analogous response was found with respect to increases in payment rates: Physicians were found to reduce the quantity of services they provided in response to higher payment rates. The results are also consistent with beneficiaries' responding to payment rate reductions by increasing their demand for physicians' services and responding to increases in payment rates by lowering their demand for physicians' services.

Of the 39.4 percent increase in the quantity of physicians' services that was observed between 1997 and 2005, most of the increase is attributable to the underlying trend in the quantity of services rather than the result of behavioral responses to changes in payment rates. Specifically, behavioral responses of physicians or beneficiaries to changes in Medicare payment rates account for only 1.4 percentage points of the 39.4 percent increase over those years, while the underlying trend increase—which captures continuing changes in medical practice over time, including the effects of changing treatment modalities and the prevalence of diseases—accounts for 38.8 percentage points of the quantity increase. (Other unexplained factors account for the remaining growth, -0.7 percent, in volume.)

PAYMENTS FOR PHYSICIANS' SERVICES

Medicare has used various methods to set payment rates for physicians' services, and to control year-to-year increases in those costs, since the program's inception. (See Box 1 for a brief history of Medicare's past efforts to control payments to physicians.) In this section of the paper, CBO describes the current method used to establish payment rates—the Medicare physician fee schedule—and how those rates are updated from year to year.

Medicare's Physician Fee Schedule: Setting Payment Rates

The Medicare physician fee schedule is used to determine payment rates for about 7,500 services provided by physicians and paid for by the Medicare program.[5] Payments are calculated in three steps.

- First, the fee schedule specifies relative value units—which measure the resources required to perform a given service—for each of three cost components:

  - Physicians' work expense, which is a measure of physicians' time and skill and the intensity of the service provided;
  - Physicians' practice expense, which is a measure of average expenses related to the maintenance of a practice, such as office rents and employees' wages;[6]
  - Physicians' malpractice cost, which is a measure of the average cost of malpractice insurance premiums.

- On average, the physicians' work expense component accounts for over 50 percent of a service's relative value, the physicians' practice expense component accounts for about 45 percent, and the malpractice expense component accounts for the remainder. The law requires that work RVUs be reviewed by the Centers for Medicare and Medicaid Services (CMS) every five years and, if necessary, revised to ensure the accuracy of payments under the fee schedule and to incorporate the changes in the resources needed to perform a service over time.[7, 8]

- Second, payment rates are adjusted to reflect regional differences in input costs. Geographic practice cost indices (GPCIs) adjust the three RVU components to account for regional differences in prices among 89 payment localities. By design, GPCIs have a national average value of 1: Areas with costs above the national average receive a GPCI greater than 1, and areas with costs below the national average receive a GPCI less than 1. Although the practice and malpractice expense GPCIs are set to fully account for regional differences, the work expense GPCI is set to reflect only a quarter of regional variations in wages. In effect, that provision limits the downward adjustment of relatively low-cost rural areas and the upward adjustment of relatively high-cost urban areas. The law requires that GPCIs be reviewed by CMS at least every three years and revised, if necessary, in a budget-neutral manner.[9]
- Third, a conversion factor translates the geographically adjusted RVUs for a given service into a dollar payment amount.

BOX 1. PAST EFFORTS TO CONTROL MEDICARE'S PAYMENTS TO PHYSICIANS

Medicare's system of payments to physicians has evolved according to a distinct chronology. When Medicare was created in 1965, the program reimbursed physicians for their services on the basis of their charges, the method of payment then used by private insurers. In addition, Medicare permitted physicians to bill beneficiaries for the amount of the charge that exceeded the amount paid by Medicare, a practice known as balance billing. However, the charge-based reimbursement system gave physicians the incentive to increase their fees from year to year to boost their revenues, and those increases led to rapid growth in Medicare's expenditures.

As concerns about the program's rising costs grew, policymakers focused on restraining those fees by relating them to the Medicare economic index (MEI). In 1972, the government mandated that annual updates to Medicare's fees for physicians' services be limited to the increase in the MEI, a provision that was implemented in 1975. Tying increases in fees to growth in the MEI was not sufficient to keep total payments from rising, however. To counter such increases in expenditures, the Congress first froze fees (from 1984 to 1986) and then raised them by amounts specified in legislation (from 1987 to 1991).

Despite those actions, spending for physicians' services continued to grow throughout the 1980s. It became apparent that limitations on the growth of physicians' fees alone—without considering the volume and intensity of services that physicians provided—was not enough to control spending. Indeed, the program's payments per physician increased almost twice as fast as did the nation's economy during the 1980s. In 1992, in response to those developments, the Congress implemented the Medicare physician fee schedule, which bases payments for individual services on measures of the relative resources used by physicians to provide their services. The implementation of the fee schedule was intended to eliminate payment differences across services and geographic areas that were unrelated to resource costs. One thing the fee schedule itself was not designed to do, however, was control spending.

In an attempt to control total spending driven by increases in the volume and intensity of physicians' services, a mechanism was also created that linked annual updates to the fee schedule to the trend in total spending relative to a target. Under that approach, the conversion factor was to be updated annually to reflect increases in physicians' costs for providing care, as measured by the MEI, and adjusted by a factor to counteract changes in the volume and intensity of services provided· per beneficiary. The first of those approaches, known as the Volume Performance Standard (VPS), established a growth rate that was determined, in part, by the historical growth in the volume and intensity of physicians' services.

The method for applying the VPS was fairly straightforward—any excess spending relative to the target triggered a reduction in the update to the fee schedule two years later. But, because the VPS system depended heavily on the historical trend in the volume and intensity of physicians' services provided to Medicare beneficiaries, it led to updates to the fee schedule that were unstable. For instance, the decline in that trend in the mid-1990s led to large increases in Medicare's payment rates for physicians' services.

Attempts to offset the budgetary effects of those increases by making successively larger cuts in payment rates further destabilized the update mechanism. Indeed, between 1992 and 1998 (the years that the VPS was in effect), the MEI varied from 2.0 percent to 3.2 percent, but the annual update to the fee schedule varied much more widely, from 0.6 percent to 7.5 percent.

Under the Balanced Budget Act of 1997, the VPS was replaced with a new volume-control mechanism that is still in effect—the Sustainable Growth Rate (SGR) system. Like the VPS, the SGR method uses a target to adjust future payment rates with the purpose of controlling growth in Medicare's expenditures for physicians' services. In contrast to the VPS, the target under the SGR mechanism is tied to growth in real (inflation-adjusted) per capita gross domestic product (GDP). The update under this approach is equal to the MEI adjusted by a factor that reflects actual spending relative to the target (measured on both an annual and a cumulative basis). (The VPS did not use cumulative spending.) Policymakers saw the SGR approach as having the advantages of objectivity and stability in comparison with the VPS. GDP growth provides an objective benchmark; moreover, changes in GDP from year to year have been considerably more stable (and generally smaller) than changes in the volume of physicians' services. Even so, updates under the SGR method have proven to be volatile as well.[1]

[1]This box is based on three sources. See Statement of Douglas Holtz-Eakin, Director, Congressional Budget Office, "Medicare's Physician Fee Schedule," before the Subcommittee on Health of the House Committee on Energy and Commerce, May 5, 2004; Government Accountability Office, *Medicare Physician Payments: Concerns About Spending Target System Prompt Interest in Considering Reforms*, GAO-05-85 (October 2004); and Congressional Research Service, *Medicare: Payments to Physicians*, CRS Report for Congress, RL31199 (updated January 2, 2007).

The above three steps are summarized in the following formula, which is used by Medicare to calculate payment rates for physicians' services under the fee schedule:

Fee schedule payment rate = conversion factor •

$$(RVU_{w.e.} \bullet GPCI_{w.e.} + RVU_{p.e.} \bullet GPCI_{p.e.} + RVU_{m.e.} \bullet GPCI_{m.e.}) , \tag{1}$$

where the subscripts denote the work expense, practice expense, and malpractice expense components. For example, in 2006 the conversion factor was \$37.8975. According to the fee schedule that year, participating physicians in New York City's borough of Manhattan received \$62.69 for each office visit made by a Medicare beneficiary. By contrast, the payment rate in Alabama for the same service was \$48.37. Similarly, treatment of a head injury in Manhattan was reimbursed at a rate of \$1,667.67 and \$1,271.93 in Alabama.[10]

In a number of circumstances, Medicare may adjust its payments for physicians' services on the basis of the characteristics of providers and other factors. For instance, nonparticipating physicians receive 95 percent of the payment established by the fee schedule. Physicians' assistants are also paid at a reduced rate, ranging from 65 percent to 85 percent of the rate allowed by the fee schedule. In addition, a number of adjustments to the fee schedule are applied to certain surgical procedures to account for variations within those procedures.[11] In an instance in which a physician submits a charge below that allowed by the fee schedule, the submitted charge becomes the actual payment rate for that service.

Consequently, the payment rate (or the allowed charge) for a service can be expressed as the fee schedule payment rate and a summary adjustment factor:

$$\text{Payment rate} = \text{Fee schedule payment rate} \cdot \text{Adjustment factor.} \qquad (2)$$

Again, the first term of the product equals the conversion factor times the adjusted RVUs. The second term represents the product of all adjustments made in each claim.[12] It should be noted that, unlike the first term of the product, this last factor is largely driven by physicians' behavior. In other words, treatment modality choices made by an individual physician can affect the payment rate for a service through the adjustment factor.

The Sustainable Growth Rate Formula: Updating Payment Rates

Annual adjustments to payment rates are computed according to the Sustainable Growth Rate formula and are carried out by updating the conversion factor. That methodology has two components: an adjustment on the basis of the MEI and a so-called update adjustment factor that accounts for differences in actual spending and expenditure targets under the SGR mechanism.

- If actual spending under the SGR does not deviate from the expenditure targets, payment rates under the physician fee schedule are simply increased by the percentage change in the price of inputs, as measured by the MEI.
- If actual spending deviates from the expenditure targets, the update adjustment factor is calculated so that, over a period of several years, cumulative spending will be brought back in line with the cumulative expenditure target. If actual spending exceeds the targets, the update adjustment factor will be negative (that is, it will reduce the amount of the increase that would otherwise occur to reflect inflation); if actual spending is less than the targets, the update adjustment factor will be positive.

Specifically, updates to payment rates are computed by multiplying the MEI and the estimated adjustment factor. For 2007, the MEI was 2.1 percent and the update adjustment factor was -7 percent. Consequently, in 2007, payment rates for physicians were scheduled to decrease by 5 percent. However, the Tax Relief and Health Care Act of 2006 overrode the formula for 2007 and held payment rates constant at their 2006 level.

Recent annual updates in Medicare payment rates have varied widely. (See Table 1 for a list of conversion factor values expressed in nominal and MEI-adjusted dollars since 1997.) In 1997, there were three separate conversion factors for primary care services, surgical services, and other nonsurgical procedures. Starting in 1998, those conversion factors were consolidated into a single conversion factor, resulting in higher payment rates in both nominal and real (MEI-adjusted) terms for primary care services and other nonsurgical procedures. From 1999 to 2001, the observed volatility tended to benefit physicians, with the conversion factor rising faster than the MEI. Since 2002, however, spending as measured by the SGR method has consistently exceeded targets established by the formula. Consequently, the conversion factor fell between 2001 and 2002. Between 2003 and 2007, lawmakers overrode the SGR mechanism, replacing negative updates with small positive or zero updates. Nevertheless, the conversionfactor did not keep up with the MEI over those years. In fact, the MEI-adjusted conversion factor in 2007 is below that of 1997.[13]

Table 1. Conversion Factors Used in Medicare's Fee Schedule for Physicians' Services, 1997 to 2007

	In Nominal Dollars		In 2006 Dollars	
	Conversion Factor	Percentage Change from Previous Year	Conversion Factor	Percentage Change from Previous Year
1997[a]	36.2410	n.a.	45.9403	n.a.
1998	36.6873	n.a.	45.4830	n.a.
1999	34.7315	-5.3	42.0679	-7.5
2000	36.6137	5.4	43.2834	2.9
2001	38.2581	4.5	44.2775	2.3
2002	36.1992	-5.4	40.8054	-7.8
2003[b]	36.7856	1.6	40.2225	-1.4
2004	37.3374	1.5	39.6419	-1.4
2005	37.8975	1.5	38.9892	-1.6
2006	37.8975	0	37.8975	-2.8
2007	37.8975	0	37.1180	-2.1

Source: Department of Health and Human Services, Centers for Medicare and Medicaid Services, "Final Rule: Medicare Program; Revisions to Payment Policies Under the Physician Fee Schedule," *Federal Register* (various years), available at www.gpoaccess.gov/fr/ index.html.

Notes: The Medicare physician fee schedule is used to determine payments for about 7,500 services provided by physicians. Payments are calculated in three steps: First, the fee schedule specifies relative value units (RVUs), which measure the resources required to perform a given service. Second, physicians' fees are adjusted to reflect regional differences in costs using geographic practice cost indices. Third, a conversion factor translates the geographically adjusted RVUs for a given service into a dollar payment amount.

n.a. = not applicable.

a. The figures displayed for 1997 are weighted averages of three separate conversion factors—primary care services ($35.7671), surgical services ($40.9603), and other nonsurgical procedures ($33.8454)—which were consolidated in 1998.

b. The conversion factor for 2003 did not become effective until March 1 of that year. Claims filed for January and February 2003 were reimbursed using the 2002 fee schedule.

TRENDS IN MEDICARE'S SPENDING FOR PHYSICIANS' SERVICES, 1997 TO 2005

Despite efforts to control costs, Medicare's spending on physicians' services has continued to increase rapidly. Between 1997 and 2005, per-beneficiary spending for physicians' services, as adjusted by the MEI, increased at an average rate of 3.8 percent per year, from $1,615 to about $2,172 in MEI-adjusted dollars, with 2006 as the base year (see Table 2).[14, 15] In contrast, per-beneficiary spending for other Medicare benefits—including coverage under Hospital Insurance (Part A) and other coverage provided under Supplemental Medical Insurance (Part B) but excluding Medicare Advantage (the program's managed care option)—grew at an average rate of 1.4 percent over the same period.[16] Except in 2002, when payment rates were reduced the most, with the conversion factor falling by 7.8 percent, the growth in Medicare's per-beneficiary spending for physicians' services, as adjusted by the MEI, has always been positive.

In the analysis that follows, recent growth in spending for physicians' services is apportioned to changes in payment rates and changes in the volume of physicians' services. The next section also discusses a number of sources that may influence the volume of physicians' services.

Table 2. Trends in Medicare's per-Beneficiary Spending for Physicians' Services, 1997 to 2005

	Per-Beneficiary Spending (In 2006 dollars)	Change from Previous Year (Percent)
1997	1,615	n.a.
1998	1,659	2.7
1999	1,711	3.1
2000	1,831	7.0
2001	1,980	8.1
2002	1,967	-0.6
2003	2,015	2.4
2004	2,126	5.5
2005	2,172	2.2
Change Between		
1997 and 2005	557	34.5

Source: Congressional Budget Office based on analysis of the Centers for Medicare and Medicaid Services' Physician Standard Analytical Files, 1997 to 2005.

Notes: Medicare's spending for physicians' services is adjusted using the Medicare economic index (MEI), with 2006 as the base year. The MEI includes changes in the cost of physicians' time and operating expenses; it is a weighted sum of the price of inputs in those two categories. Changes in "all-factor" productivity are also incorporated into the index as a way of accounting for improvements in physicians' productivity.

Spending includes both Medicare's share of fees and that paid by beneficiaries through cost sharing (in the form of deductibles and copayments).

n.a. = not applicable.

CBO's Decomposition Analysis

This section describes the data sources and methodology that CBO used and presents decomposition results of the determinants of per-beneficiary physician spending between

1997 and 2005. More specifically, the decomposition analysis quantifies the impact of changes in payment rates and changes in the volume of physicians' services on the growth in Medicare's spending for those services.

Data Sources

The data set used in this analysis is constructed by combining Medicare claims for physicians' services and demographic data on beneficiaries with payment rates from the Medicare fee schedule. The analysis is based on data from 1997 to 2005. The resulting nine-year sample consists of roughly 2.7 million beneficiaries, with an average of approximately 300,000 beneficiaries per year and 27 procedures per beneficiary per year.

Medicare claims data for physicians' services are obtained from the Physician Standard Analytical Files (SAFs) compiled by CMS. The SAFs contain final-action (nonrejected) claims for physicians' services for a 1 percent sample of Medicare beneficiaries enrolled in the fee-for-service sector of the program. The data consist of detailed claims information on procedures, payments, and providers, including the type of procedure, or Healthcare Common Procedure Coding System code; the submitted charge; Medicare's allowed charge; the site of treatment; the provider type and specialty; and the provider's carrier number and locality code.[17]

Claims data are merged with the Medicare Denominator file, which includes basic demographic characteristics, such as each beneficiary's age, sex, race, and, if applicable, date of death. Each claim is further augmented with data from the fee schedule. The fee schedule, which is updated annually, lists all procedures covered by Medicare as well as the procedures' corresponding RVUs, and the conversion factor.[18] Lastly, GPCIs are added to each claim, using the carrier number and locality code.[19]

Methodology

As stated in equations (1) and (2), payment rates governed by the fee schedule are calculated as the product of the conversion factor, the sum of the three RVU components adjusted by their corresponding GPCIs, and a summary adjustment factor. By separating the different components that make up the payment rate for each service provided by a physician, CBO's analysis can assess the importance of each component in explaining recent spending growth for physicians' services.

The effect of changes in prices and in the quantity of services on spending growth can be calculated by computing a decomposition of that growth into portions attributable to each of the two elements.[20] Specifically, changes in spending between years t and $t + 1$ are expressed as follows:

$$
\begin{aligned}
P^{t+1} \bullet Q^{t+1} - P^t \bullet Q^t &= (P^{t+1} \bullet Q^{t+1} - P^{t+1} \bullet Q^t) + (P^{t+1} \bullet Q^t - P^t \bullet Q^t) \\
&= P^{t+1} \bullet (Q^{t+1} - Q^t) + (P^{t+1} - P^t) \bullet Q^t \\
&= P^{t+1} \bullet \Delta Q + \Delta P \bullet Q^t,
\end{aligned}
\tag{3}
$$

where t denotes the year, which ranges from 1997 to 2004.[21, 22]

The first term in the decomposition captures changes in spending that are attributable to changes in quantity (or volume and intensity) and equals the difference in spending between years t and $t + 1$, holding prices (or payment rates) constant. The second term accounts for changes in spending that are attributable to changes in prices. This term requires calculating what spending would have been in year $t + 1$ had quantities remained at year t levels.[23]

In order to isolate how the individual components of Medicare's prices affect spending, the above decomposition is modified as follows:

$$
\begin{aligned}
P^{t+1} \bullet Q^{t+1} - P^t \bullet Q^t &= CF^{t+1} \bullet RVU^{t+1} \bullet adj^{t+1} \bullet Q^{t+1} - CF^t \bullet RVU^t \bullet adj^t \bullet Q^t \\
&= (CF^{t+1} - CF^t) \bullet RVU^t \bullet adj^t \bullet Q^t + CF^{t+1} \bullet (RVU^{t+1} - RVU^t) \bullet adj^t \bullet Q^t + \\
&\quad CF^{t+1} \bullet RVU^{t+1} \bullet (adj^{t+1} - adj^t) \bullet Q^t + CF^{t+1} \bullet RVU^{t+1} \bullet adj^{t+1} \bullet (Q^{t+1} - Q^t) \qquad (4) \\
&= \Delta CF \bullet RVU^t \bullet adj^t \bullet Q^t + CF^{t+1} \bullet \Delta RVU \bullet adj^t \bullet Q^t + CF^{t+1} \bullet RVU^{t+1} \bullet \Delta adj \bullet Q^t + \\
&\quad CF^{t+1} \bullet RVU^{t+1} \bullet adj^{t+1} \bullet \Delta Q,
\end{aligned}
$$

where CF represents the conversion factor; RVU is the sum of all RVU components adjusted by their respective GPCIs; adj is the adjustment factor; and Q is quantity of services. The first term corresponds to the share of spending growth explained by changes in the conversion factor. The other terms represent the share of spending growth attributable to changes in RVUs, changes in the adjustment factor, and changes in the quantity of physicians' services provided.

Results

Table 3 and Table 4 summarize the results from the separate decompositions. Table 3 presents the results of a decomposition of the observed increase in spending for physicians' services into a fraction that can be attributed to changes in payment rates and a fraction that can be attributed to changes in the volume of physicians' services; Table 4 explores how changes in the components of payment rates affect that growth in spending.

Applying the decomposition to spending on physicians' services suggests that changes in the quantities of those services fully account for changes in spending between 1997 and 2005 (see Table 3). Changes in the quantity of physicians' services alone would have increased spending by 39.4 percent. A smaller reduction in payment rates (4.9 percent) offsets a portion of that increase, resulting in a net increase in spending of 34.5 percent.

Whereas the effect of changes in the quantity of services on spending was always positive over the sample years (ranging from 1.5 percent between 1997 and 1998 to 6.6 percent between 2001 and 2002), the effect of changes in prices on spending was considerably more variable (ranging from -7.2 percent in between 2001 and 2002 to 3.8 percent between 1999 and 2000.) Except for the 2001–2002 period, changes in the quantity of services more than compensated for any declines in prices, resulting in positive spending growth in all but that one year.

Focusing next on the individual components of payment rates, the results indicate that updates to the conversion factor between 1997 and 2005 would have resulted in a 14.1 percent reduction in spending had the adjusted RVUs, the adjustment factor, and the quantity of physicians' services remained at 1997 levels (see Table 4). In most years, changes in

RVUs explain only a small portion of the overall change in spending. That is as expected because most RVU changes were intended to have a negligible impact on spending. An exception occurred in 1999, when CMS eliminated a temporary adjustment factor to RVUs, which had effectively reduced physician work expense RVUs by 8.3 percent.[24] So removing that adjustment amounted to an increase in RVUs in 1999 as compared to 1998 levels. Also, in 2004, the Medicare Prescription Drug Improvement and Modernization Act of 2003 established a floor of 1.0 in the GPCI work component, effectively increasing adjusted RVUs between 2003 and 2004. Lastly, the adjustment factor played a negligible role in explaining spending changes, accounting for 2 percent (0.7 percent of the 34.5 percent) of the estimated increase in spending between 1997 and 2005.

Table 3. Decomposition of Changes in Medicare's per-Beneficiary Spending for Physicians' Services, 1997 to 2005

(Percent)	Change in Spending Attributable to:		
	Changes in the Price of Services	**Changes in the Quantity of Services**	**Change in Per-Beneficiary Spending**
1997 to 1998	1.2	1.5	2.7
1998 to 1999	-0.6	3.7	3.1
1999 to 2000	3.8	3.2	7.0
2000 to 2001	2.2	6.0	8.1
2001 to 2002	-7.2	6.6	-0.6
2002 to 2003	-1.9	4.3	2.4
2003 to 2004	0.9	4.5	5.5
2004 to 2005	-1.8	4.0	2.2
Change Between			
1997 and 2005	-4.9	39.4	34.5

Source: Congressional Budget Office based on analysis of the Centers for Medicare and Medicaid Services' Physician Standard Analytical Files, 1997 to 2005.

Notes: Medicare's spending for physicians' services is adjusted using the Medicare economic index (MEI), with 2006 as the base year. The MEI includes changes in the cost of physicians' time and operating expenses; it is a weighted sum of the price of inputs in those two categories. Changes in "all-factor" productivity are also incorporated into the index as a way of accounting for improvements in physicians' productivity.

Spending includes both Medicare's share of fees and that paid by beneficiaries through cost sharing (in the form of deductibles and copayments).

In CBO's analysis, "price" refers to Medicare's allowed charge for a given service. "Quantity" refers to the volume and intensity of services provided.

Components may not add to totals because of rounding.

In this specification, the change in spending that is attributable to changes in the conversion factor and to changes in RVUs may be interpreted as the share of spending growth attributable to changes in the components of payment rates that are exogenous to physicians. Changes in the conversion factor and RVUs cannot explain the observed growth in physician spending between 1997 and 2005. It should be noted that the analysis in Table 4 captures the extent to which changes in prices directly affect spending but not their indirect effect through changes in the level of physicians' services. As previously discussed, physicians may respond to changes in prices by adjusting the quantity of services they provide, and beneficiaries by adjusting the quantity they demand. Therefore, the estimated impact of changes in the quantity of physicians' services reported in Table 4 may be driven in part by changes in prices.

Table 4. Expanded Decomposition of Changes in Medicare's per-Beneficiary Spending for Physicians' Services, 1997 to 2005

(Percent)	Change in Spending Attributable to Changes in the Components of Price					
	Overall	Conversion Factor	RVUs[a]	Adjustment Factor	Change in Spending Attributable to Changes in the Quantity of Services	Change in Per-Beneficiary Spending
1997 to 1998	1.2	0.2	0.5	0.6	1.5	2.7
1998 to 1999	-0.6	-7.5	7.0	-0.1	3.7	3.1
1999 to 2000	3.8	2.9	0.3	0.6	3.2	7.0
2000 to 2001	2.2	2.3	0.1	-0.2	6.0	8.1
2001 to 2002	-7.2	-7.8	0.3	0.3	6.6	-0.6
2002 to 2003	-1.9	-1.6	-0.2	-0.1	4.3	2.4
2003 to 2004	0.9	-1.4	2.1	0.3	4.5	5.5
2004 to 2005	-1.8	-1.6	-0.3	0.2	4.0	2.2
Change Between						
1997 and 2005	-4.9	-14.1	8.5	0.7	39.4	34.5

Source: Congressional Budget Office based on analysis of the Centers for Medicare and Medicaid Services' Physician Standard Analytical Files, 1997 to 2005.

Notes: The Medicare physician fee schedule is used to determine payments for about 7,500 services provided by physicians. Payments are calculated in three steps: First, the fee schedule specifies relative value units (RVUs), which measure the resources required to perform a given service. Second, physicians' fees are adjusted to reflect regional differences in costs using geographic practice cost indices. Third, a conversion factor translates the geographically adjusted RVUs for a given service into a dollar payment amount.

Medicare's spending for physicians' services is adjusted using the Medicare economic index (MEI), with 2006 as the base year. The MEI includes changes in the cost of physicians' time and operating expenses; it is a weighted sum of the price of inputs in those two categories. Changes in "all-factor" productivity are also incorporated into the index as a way of accounting for improvements in physicians' productivity.

Spending includes both Medicare's share of fees and that paid by beneficiaries through cost sharing (in the form of deductibles and copayments).

In CBO's analysis, "price" refers to Medicare's allowed charge for a given service. "Quantity" refers to the volume and intensity of services provided.

Components may not add to totals because of rounding.

a. In this analysis, "RVUs" refer to geographically adjusted RVUs.

Discussion

The decomposition results suggest that changes in the quantity of services are largely responsible for changes in spending for physicians' services between 1997 and 2005. Consequently, it is useful to examine the underlying reasons for the increase in the volume of physicians' services. Those factors include the secular trend in spending for physicians' services, behavioral responses to changes in payment rates, and changes in market conditions.[25]

Secular Trend in Spending

Recent research has shown that a key determinant of the underlying upward trend in spending for medical care is an increase in the use of medical services. In particular, increases in the prevalence of diseases and medical innovation as well as changes in treatment modalities have been major contributors to spending growth.[26] The estimate of the secular trend in the empirical analyses in the next section includes the impact of changes in the demographic characteristics of beneficiaries and in the volume of services—both existing and newly covered services— covered by Medicare.

Changes in the demographic characteristics of the Medicare fee-for-service population can affect the volume of services provided by physicians because the use of medical services varies across different demographic groups. For example, the volume of services may increase if the composition of beneficiaries shifts toward groups (such as older beneficiaries) that use more services. Over the nine-year period analyzed in this paper, the demographic composition of the population changed only slightly. The percentage of beneficiaries that were 65 years old and younger increased, while the percentage of beneficiaries ages 65 to 74 decreased. There was a small shift toward nonwhite beneficiaries and male beneficiaries and a lower prevalence of beneficiaries who died during the year. (Table A-2 in the appendix presents demographic characteristics of the sample in 1997 and 2005; Table A-3 shows average monthly spending on the basis of demographic characteristics for the same years.) CBO's analysis shows that demographic changes had a negligible impact on the growth in spending between 1997 and 2005. More specifically, had the demographic composition of beneficiaries remained at 1997 levels, MEI-adjusted per-beneficiary spending in 2005 would have been $2,135 rather than $2,172, the level of actual spending.[27, 28]

Changes in the services covered by Medicare can also affect the volume of services that physicians provide. That is, changes in spending are partly determined by the addition of both newly covered services (such as colorectal cancer screening and pelvic examinations, which were added to the list of Medicare covered services by the Balanced Budget Act of 1997) and new medical treatments. A comparison of actual Medicare spending on physicians' services over the 1997–2005 period with spending that included only those physicians' services available in 1997 suggests that new and newly covered services may explain some of the increase in Medicare spending over that period. In fact, per-enrollee MEI-adjusted physician spending growth between 1997 and 2005 is 18.6 percent when including only physicians' services that were covered by Medicare in 1997, compared with growth of 34.5 percent for all services— those covered in 1997 and any newly covered services in 1998 to 2005—as reported above. (See Table A-4 in the appendix for these estimates.) It should be emphasized that estimating the impact of new services on spending for physicians' services is challenging because relying on additions to the Medicare physician fee schedule to identify that effect may lead to both overestimates and underestimates. The impact of new and newly covered services is overestimated to the extent that new service codes replace old ones. By contrast, this impact is underestimated when new and newly covered services operate within old service codes.[29]

Behavioral Impact of Changes in Payment Rates

The observed increases in spending that are attributable to changes in the quantity of physicians' services may also be affected by changes in Medicare's fee schedule to the extent that beneficiaries and physicians respond to changes in payment rates. Physicians may respond to changes in those rates by adjusting the quantity of services supplied. In addition, the demand for physicians' services may also vary with changes in payment rates because beneficiaries are financially responsible for a portion of the payment rate in the form of cost sharing. Given the significant changes in payment rates to physicians over the 1997–2005 period, that so-called volume offset could account for some share of the change in Medicare's spending.

Marketwide Conditions

Although the analysis that follows cannot account for changes in marketwide conditions because of data limitations, those variations may also partially explain the observed changes in Medicare's spending for physicians' services. Specifically, the volume of spending for physicians' services may be influenced by changes in market-level characteristics, such as shifts in the level of enrollment in health maintenance organizations (HMOs) and changing rates of reimbursements made by private payers.

Medicare's HMO enrollment rates increased steadily in the 1990s, rising from 4 percent in 1990 to 16 percent in 2000. However, enrollment declined between 2000 and 2003 but then rose again between 2003 and 2004.[30] Changes in enrollment in Medicare HMOs could result in changes in the characteristics of beneficiaries in the fee-for-service population and, therefore, could affect spending for physicians' services. In addition, because the cost containment features of HMOs tend to steer physicians toward a specific practice style, changes in HMO enrollment could influence the volume of services they provide to Medicare patients.

Changes in physicians' payment rates in the private-payer market can also affect Medicare's spending for physicians' services by altering relative profit margins. Assuming that physicians are able to substitute privately insured patients for Medicare patients, changes in private fees may have an effect on Medicare spending. For example, in years when Medicare payment rates fall relative to those rates paid by private insurers, physicians may choose to shift away from Medicare patients to privately insured patients in order to reduce income losses. Private claims data are not widely available, but there is some evidence that, on average, the ratio of Medicare to private-payer fees has grown from about 70 percent in 1996 to roughly 83 percent in 2005.[31]

The next section presents the mechanisms by which changes in payment rates can elicit changes in volume or behavioral responses and reviews the research examining that effect.

Then, a methodology is introduced that aims to measure the secular trend in spending for physicians' services and to determine the degree to which behavioral responses to changes in payment rates account for the observed growth in Medicare spending for physicians' services.

THE EFFECTS OF CHANGES IN PAYMENT RATES ON THE VOLUME OF PHYSICIANS' SERVICES: EXISTING EVIDENCE

There are two paths by which the volume of physicians' services could be affected by recent changes in payment rates:

- First, because beneficiaries generally pay 20 percent of the approved amount for covered services (in excess of the annual deductible), changes in payment rates directly affect beneficiaries' out-of-pocket costs. Thus, patients may demand more care when physicians' payment rates are reduced because their cost sharing (in the form of deductibles and copayments) is lower, and vice versa.[32]
- Second, physicians may respond to changes in payment rates by adjusting the supply of services they provide to Medicare beneficiaries. Under a standard economic model that treats the physician as a profit-maximizing firm, a decline in payment rates leads to a decline in the quantity of services provided; increases in payment rates have the opposite effect. An alternative model incorporates the notion that, in response to lower payment rates, physicians may exert influence over the demand for their services in order to replace some or all of their lost income; analogously, they may reduce the quantity of their services if payment rates increase.[33] (That phenomenon is termed demand inducement.) The effect of a reduction in payment rates on the volume of physicians' services depends on the relative size of the "income effect" and the "substitution effect." The income effect generates a volume offset, as physicians compensate for their loss in income by increasing the volume of services they provide. The substitution effect, in contrast, results in decreasing volume, as physicians substitute (relatively higher paying) private-payer patients for Medicare patients. This effect is magnified to the extent that physicians are able to substitute nonwork activities (or leisure) for labor. Thus, when the income effect dominates the substitution effect, reductions in payments rates would be expected to result in an increase in the supply of physicians' services. Conversely, in cases in which the substitution effect is larger than the income effect, reductions in payment rates would be expected to result in a decline in the volume of physicians' services.

Studies that evaluate behavioral responses to changes in Medicare payment rates typically focus on three key empirical questions: What is the direction of the behavioral response? What is the magnitude of that response? And, is the response similar for decreases and increases in payment rates? (In other words, is the behavioral response symmetric?) A number of studies attempt to answer those questions by analyzing certain sets of medical procedures that have been affected by changes in payment rates. In general, the studies estimate elasticities based on regression analyses of changes in the quantity of services provided on changes in the prices of those services.[34] (Elasticities measure the sensitivity of the volume of physicians' services to changes in payment rates for those services.)

Previous studies of the effects of changes in Medicare payment rates on the level of services that physicians provide yield mixed evidence of a behavioral response. Those studies can be divided into two categories:

- More recent studies generally tend to explicitly follow a framework developed by Thomas McGuire and Mark Pauly—in their *Journal of Health Economics* paper— by estimating a supply function as suggested by the theoretical model. This line of research has been more likely to find a positive relationship between changes in payment rates and changes in the volume of services provided.[35]

- Older empirical studies tend to find that physicians respond to reductions in payment rates by increasing the volume of their services, with elasticities ranging from −0.2 to −0.4.[36] In other words, a 1 percent reduction in payment rates would lead to a 0.2 percent to 0.4 percent increase in the volume of services provided. Some studies also show that certain specialties are more likely or better able to respond to changes in payment rates. In general, surgery appears to be the most responsive to such changes. One study estimated an elasticity of -0.83 for surgical specialty groups.[37,38]

Among those studies that find a negative relationship between changes in payment rates and changes in the volume of services, evidence on the symmetry of the volume response is mixed. For example, one study found no evidence of asymmetric responses, leading the authors to conclude that the volume response is symmetric.[39] In contrast, a study by CMS's Office of the Actuary concluded that physicians respond asymmetrically to changes in payment rates. In particular, that study found a statistically significant positive volume response to price decreases of 31 percent ($p < 0.05$) and a negative response of 13 percent to increases in payment rates, although the latter estimate was not statistically different from zero ($p = 0.35$).[40] On the basis of those findings, CMS adjusted its estimate of the volume offset downward, from 50 percent to 30 percent, for reductions in payment rates only. In the case of increases, CMS has continued to assume no volume offset.

The analysis that follows estimates the impact of a behavioral response in conjunction with the underlying trend in the volume of physicians' services on changes in spending. The behavioral response is regarded from a systemwide perspective, with a focus on the budgetary implications of changes in payment rates for physicians' services due to that response. For this purpose, the manner in which a new level of services or spending is realized is not the key question addressed here. That is, the analysis does not attempt to identify the source of the behavioral response (to the extent that such a response exists).

CBO'S REGRESSION ANALYSIS

When evaluating policy proposals related to changes in Medicare payment rates for physicians' services, the Congressional Budget Office projects spending on the basis of assumptions regarding the secular trend in spending for physicians' services and any behavioral response that accompanies changes in payment rates. Toward that end, this section attempts to distinguish the underlying trend over time in the quantity of physicians' services from the changes in services that result from behavioral responses to changes in Medicare's payment rates. It should be emphasized that the analysis does not attempt to identify the individual determinants of volume growth as discussed in the previous section. Instead, it aims to validate a range of estimates for the secular trend in spending for physicians' services and the behavioral response to changes in payment rates consistent with recent changes in the fee schedule and spending.

Table 5. Summary of Regressions of Medicare's Actual per-Beneficiary Spending on Predicted per-Beneficiary Spending

Predicted Spending	Actual Spending per Beneficiary	
	Model 1: Impose Symmetric Behavioral Responses	Model 2: Allow for Asymmetric Behavioral Responses
Trend in Quantity of Services	1.042 *	1.036 *
Provided (1 + G)	(0.005)	(0.008)
	[1.030, 1.054]	[1.014, 1.058]
Behavioral Response	-0.279	n.a.
	(0.150)	
	[-0.647, 0.088]	
Behavioral Response to Increases in Payment Rates	n.a.	0.113[a]
		(0.465)
		[-1.083, 1.309]
Behavioral Response to Decreases in Payment Rates	n.a.	-0.434
		(0.231)
		[-1.029, 0.161]
R^2	0.99	0.99

Source: Congressional Budget Office based on analysis of the Centers for Medicare and Medicaid Services' Physician Standard Analytical Files, 1997 to 2005.

Notes: Medicare's spending for physicians' services is adjusted using the Medicare economic index (MEI), with 2006 as the base year. The MEI includes changes in the cost of physicians' time and operating expenses; it is a weighted sum of the price of inputs in those two categories.

Changes in "all-factor" productivity are also incorporated into the index as a way of accounting for improvements in physicians' productivity.

Spending includes both Medicare's share of fees and that paid by beneficiaries through cost sharing (in the form of deductibles and copayments).

Under the assumption of symmetric behavior (Model 1), physicians and beneficiaries are constrained to exhibit similar volume response to either payment rate increases or decreases. The asymmetric response assumption (Model 2) allows for differing behavioral responses to both positive and negative changes in payment rates.

Estimated standard errors appear in parentheses. Estimated 95 percent confidence intervals appear in brackets.

*=$p < 0.01$

n.a. = not applicable.

a. This estimate implies that an increase in Medicare's payment rates to physicians is associated. with an increase in spending of a greater percentage than the increase in payment rates.

Methodology

The approach uses data that are added up to the national level—the same level of aggregation that is used for budget projections of spending on physicians' services and for evaluations of the budgetary consequences of changing the update factor for physicians' payment rates.[41] Specifically, the analysis finds the values of the secular trend and the behavioral response that minimize the sum of the squares error of the difference between actual and predicted spending. Predicted spending in year $t + 1$ is given by:

$$\text{Predicted spending}^{t+1} = (1+G) \bullet P^{t+1} \bullet Q^t + R \bullet (P^{t+1} \bullet Q^t - P^t \bullet Q^t), \qquad (5)$$

where $(1 + G)$ represents the secular trend in the quantity of services that are provided by physicians and R is the behavioral response parameter for changes in Medicare's payment rates. The first term captures predicted spending in period $t + 1$, with payment rates updated according to the fee schedule in year $t + 1$ and quantities increased by a trend factor $(1 + G)$. The second term captures the behavioral response to changes in payment rates. This response, R, is based on changes in payment rates between years t and $t + 1$.

Solving this minimization problem is equivalent to estimating an ordinary least squares regression, where the dependent variable is actual spending in year $t + 1$ and the independent variables are given by the predicted spending specification in equation (5). The regressions include two specifications. In the first specification (Model 1), the behavioral response is constrained to be the same for both ductions and increases in payment rates—a symmetric response. In a second specification (Model 2), the symmetry restriction is relaxed, and the behavioral response is allowed to differ according to whether payment rates increase or decrease.[42] (See Table 5 for estimates of the quantity trend (G) and the behavioral response (R).)[43]

Results

Two key findings are illustrated in Table 5: The minimization problem identifies a sizable positive underlying trend in the use of physicians' services, and it indicates that changes in payment rates appear to affect the behavior of physicians and/or beneficiaries. The estimate of the secular trend in the quantity of services ranges from 3.6 percent to 4.2 percent and is statistically significant in both models. In Model 1, where the behavioral response is assumed to be symmetric, the response coefficient equals -0.279 ($P = 0.11$). In other words, a change in payment rates that would increase or decrease spending by $1,000 would be potentially offset by a change in the quantity of services provided that would yield a corresponding decrease or increase in spending of roughly $280. That estimate falls within the range of estimates of the previous literature that finds a behavioral response.[44]

In Model 2, where the behavioral response is allowed to vary according to whether payment rates are expected to increase or decrease, the separate estimates of the behavioral responses are 0.113 for increases in payment rates (P = 0.82) and -0.434 for decreases (P = 0.12), potentially indicating an asymmetric response. The lack of precision in the estimates (as indicated by the large standard errors) is such that neither is E. statistically different from zero. Moreover, a frequently used statistical test (an F-test) cannot reject the equality of the two parameters (symmetry).[45]

**Table 6. Summary of the Effect of Changes in the Prices and Quantity of Physicians'
Services on Medicare's per-Beneficiary Spending, 1997 to 2005**

(Percent)	Change in Spending Attributable to Changes in the Components of Price				Change in Spending Attributable to Changes in the Quantity of Services				
	Overall	Conversion Factor	RVUs[a]	Adjustment Factor	Overall	Secular Trend[b]	Behavioral Response[b]	Residual[b]	Change in per-Benefici-ary Spending
1997 to 1998	1.2	0.2	0.5	0.6	1.5	4.2	-0.3	-2.3	2.7
1998 to 1999	-0.6	-7.5	7.0	-0.1	3.7	4.2	0.2	-0.6	3.1
1999 to 2000	3.8	2.9	0.3	0.6	3.2	4.2	-1.1	0.0	7.0
2000 to 2001	2.2	2.3	0.1	-0.2	6.0	4.2	-0.6	2.4	8.1
2001 to 2002	-7.2	-7.8	0.3	0.3	6.6	4.2	2.0	0.4	-0.6
2002 to 2003	-1.9	-1.6	-0.2	-0.1	4.3	4.2	0.5	-0.4	2.4
2003 to 2004	0.9	-1.4	2.1	0.3	4.5	4.2	-0.3	0.6	5.2
2004 to 2005	-1.8	-1.6	-0.3	0.2	4.0	4.2	0.5	-0.7	2.2
Change Between									
1997 and 2005	-4.9	-14.1	8.5	0.7	39.4	38.8	1.4	-0.7	34.5

Source: Congressional Budget Office based on analysis of the Centers for Medicare and Medicaid Services' Physician Standard Analytical Files, 1997 to 2005.

Notes: The Medicare physician fee schedule is used to determine payments for about 7,500 services provided by physicians. Payments are calculated in three steps: First, the fee schedule specifies relative value units (RVUs), which measure the resources required to perform a given service. Second, physicians' fees are adjusted to reflect regional differences in costs using geographic practice cost indices. Third, a conversion factor translates the geographically adjusted RVUs for a given service into a dollar payment amount.

Medicare's spending for physicians' services is adjusted using the Medicare economic index (MEI), with 2006 as the base year. The MEI includes changes in the cost of physicians' time and operating expenses; it is a weighted sum of the price of inputs in those two categories. Changes in "all-factor" productivity are also incorporated into the index as a way of accounting for improvements in physicians' productivity.

Spending includes both Medicare's share of fees and that paid by beneficiaries through cost sharing (in the form of deductibles and copayments).

In CBO's analysis, "price" refers to Medicare's allowed charge for a given service. "Quantity" refers to the volume and intensity of services provided.

Components may not add to totals because of rounding.

a. In this analysis, "RVUs" refer to geographically adjusted RVUs.

b. Estimates from the empirical (symmetric) model are used to distinguish the effect of the separate components of changes in quantities on changes in spending. The secular trend captures changes in spending due to increases in the use of medical services. The behavioral response measures the effect of a change in payment rates in the behavior of physicians and beneficiaries. The residual captures unexplained factors including errors in measuring spending that cause the empirical model to fall short of explaining all of the changes in physician spending over time.

Although those estimates of the behavioral response are consistent with other published estimates, the analysis is limited in three ways. First, even when the analysis encompasses more years than previous studies do, it is still based on only nine years of data. Second, the lack of data on private fees precludes an examination of their potential impact on Medicare's spending for physicians' services.[46] Lastly, one question that cannot be answered by this analysis is whether the observed behavioral response is driven by physicians' responses or by those of beneficiaries.[47]

Discussion

The results presented in Table 5 can be used to estimate the separate effects of the underlying trend in the volume of services provided and the behavioral response on spending growth. Those estimates are calculated by applying the regression point estimates from Model 1 in Table 5 to the decomposition analysis above (based on equation (4)). The results, shown in Table 6, indicate that the secular trend in volume explains the vast majority of the change in spending attributable to changes in quantity. The impact of behavioral responses to changes in payment rates on spending is much smaller in size and reaches its highest value in the 2001–2002 period, when payment rates were reduced the most. The residual source of change in quantity affecting spending is also small. That residual captures unexplained factors including errors in the measuring of spending that cause the empirical model to fall short of explaining all of the changes in spending for physicians' services over time.

CONCLUSION

CBO's analysis shows that the recent growth in per-beneficiary Medicare expenditures for physicians' services, as adjusted by the MEI, can be largely explained by increases in the volume and intensity of services provided. The analysis estimates a positive annual trend of about 4 percent in the volume and intensity of physicians' services. Notwithstanding the overall growth in physician spending over the 1997–2005 period, the conversion factor—the main mechanism that determines changes in Medicare's payment rates for physicians' services—actually declined by 14 percent over that period (in MEI-adjusted dollars).

An additional question is whether changes in payment rates affect spending indirectly through a so-called behavioral response. The empirical analysis presented here suggests a behavioral response of roughly 28 percent (symmetric) in a direction opposite to the change in payment rates (decreases in payment rates are associated with increases in volume, and increases in payment rates are associated with decreases in volume), which is consistent with the range of estimates of the previous literature. In explaining changes in spending, however, the behavioral response accounts for only a small fraction of that change—1.4 percentage points of the 34.5 percent increase in spending).

It is unclear whether the estimated behavioral response will apply in the future, as the projected cuts in payment rates may be significantly different from those on which this analysis is based. That is, the estimated behavioral response shown in this paper is based on payment rates varying from year to year and changing in different directions, but future changes—if the SGR mechanism is followed—are expected to persist in the direction of reducing payment rates, which could lead to behavioral responses that are qualitatively and quantitatively different.

APPENDIX

The tables in this appendix offer background statistics supporting the Congressional Budget Office's analysis.

Table A.1. Trends in Medicare's Spending for Physicians' Services and in Program Enrollment, 1997 to 2005

	Spending		Enrollment	
	Total pending (Billions of 2006 dollars)	Percentage Change from Previous Year	Number of Beneficiaries (Millions)	Percentage Change from Previous Year
1997	50.5	n.a.	31.2	n.a.
1998	50.6	0.3	30.5	-2.4
1999	51.5	1.9	30.1	-1.2
2000	55.6	7.8	30.4	0.8
2001	61.9	11.3	31.2	2.9
2002	63.5	2.7	32.3	3.4
2003	66.7	5.0	33.1	2.4
2004	71.4	7.0	33.6	1.5
2005	73.4	2.8	33.8	0.6

Source: Congressional Budget Office based on analysis (for spending) of the Centers for Medicare and Medicaid Services' Physician Standard Analytical Files, 1997 to 2005, and on enrollment figures from that agency's Office of the Actuary.

Notes: Medicare's spending for physicians' services is adjusted using the Medicare economic index (MEI), with 2006 as the base year. The MEI includes changes in the cost of physicians' time and operating expenses; it is a weighted sum of the price of inputs in those two categories. Changes in "all-factor" productivity are also incorporated into the index as a way of accounting for improvements in physicians' productivity.

Spending includes both Medicare's share of payment rates and that paid by beneficiaries through cost sharing (in the form of deductibles and copayments).

n.a. = not applicable.

Table A.2. Demographic Characteristics of Medicare Beneficiaries, 1997 and 2005

(Percent)		
	1997	**2005**
Age		
Under 65	14.8	18.6
65 to 74	43.8	39.9
75 to 84	30.8	30.3
85 and over	10.7	11.3
Race		
Black	8.6	9.5
Other	4.5	5.1
White	86.9	85.4
Sex		
Female	59.3	58.2
Male	40.7	41.8
Death Occurred		
During Year		
No	93.7	94.1
Yes	6.3	5.9

Source: Congressional Budget Office based on analysis of the Centers for Medicare and Medicaid Services' Physician Standard Analytical Files and Denominator Files, 1997 and 2005.

Note: Percentages in each category may not add to 100 percent because of rounding.

Table A.3. Medicare's per-Beneficiary Monthly Spending for Physicians' Services, by Program Participants' Demographic Characteristics, 1997 and 2005

(Dollars)		
	1997	**2005**
Age		
Under 65	165	205
65 to 74	150	194
75 to 84	184	241
85 and over	186	230
Race		
Black	185	225
Other	181	228
White	164	212
Sex		
Female	157	208
Male	179	223
Death Occurred		
During Year		
No	137	185
Yes	592	683

Source: Congressional Budget Office based on analysis of the Centers for Medicare and Medicaid
  Services' Physician Standard Analytical Files and Denominator Files, 1997 and 2005.

Notes: Medicare's spending for physicians' services is adjusted using the Medicare economic index
  (MEI), with 2006 as the base year. The MEI includes changes in the cost of physicians' time and
  operating expenses; it is a weighted sum of the price of inputs in those two categories. Changes in
  "all-factor" productivity are also incorporated into the index as a way of accounting for
  improvements in physicians' productivity.

  Spending includes both Medicare's share of payment rates and that paid by beneficiaries through
  cost sharing (in the form of deductibles and copayments).

Table A.4. Impact of Changes in Covered Services on Medicare's per-Beneficiary Spending, 1997 to 2005

(Dollars)	All Services	Services Covered in 1997	Percentage of Total	New Services Available After 1997	Percentage of Total
1997	1,615	1,615	100	0	0
1998	1,659	1,616	97	43	3
1999	1,711	1,657	97	54	3
2000	1,831	1,749	96	81	4
2001	1,980	1,874	95	106	5
2002	1,967	1,836	93	132	7
2003	2,015	1,867	93	149	7
2004	2,126	1,926	91	200	9
2005	2,172	1,916	88	257	12

Source: Congressional Budget Office based on analysis of the Centers for Medicare and Medicaid
  Services' Physician Standard Analytical Files, 1997 to 2005.

Notes: Medicare's spending for physicians' services is adjusted using the Medicare economic index
  (MEI), with 2006 as the base year. The MEI includes changes in the cost of physicians' time and
  operating expenses; it is a weighted sum of the price of inputs in those two categories. Changes in
  "all-factor" productivity are also incorporated into the index as a way of accounting for
  improvements in physicians' productivity.

  Spending includes both Medicare's share of payment rates and that paid by beneficiaries through
  cost sharing (in the form of deductibles and copayments).

  · The category "Services Covered in 1997" refers to services eligible for reimbursement that year
  under Medicare's physician fee schedule. After 1997, the fee schedule was expanded to include
  additional services.

End Notes

[1] For a more detailed discussion of the SGR mechanism, see Congressional Budget Office, *The Sustainable Growth Rate Formula for Setting Medicare's Physician Payment Rates*, CBO Economic and Budget Issue Brief (September 6, 2006).

[2] The Medicare economic index measures changes in the cost of physicians' time and operating expenses; it is a weighted sum of the prices of inputs in those two categories. Most of the components of the index come from the Bureau of Labor Statistics. Changes in the cost of physicians' time are measured using changes in nonfarm labor costs. Changes in "all-factor" productivity are also incorporated into the index as a way of accounting for improvements in physicians' productivity. The productivity adjustment to the MEI reduces its rate of growth.

[3] Between 1997 and 2005, the MEI rose by 23 percent, and enrollment in Medicare Part B grew by 8 percent. Together, those changes accounted for about 40 percent of the change in total spending during that period.

[4] "Intensity" refers to the complexity of services utilized in delivering patient care. For example, use of a computerized axial tomography (CAT) scan rather than an x-ray would represent an increase in intensity.

[5] The fee schedule is also used for services provided by certain nonphysician practitioners (such as physicians' assistants and nurse practitioners) and limited licensed practitioners (such as chiropractors, podiatrists, and optometrists).

[6] Certain services are assigned separate practice expense RVUs on the basis of whether or not the services are provided at a "nonfacility" (for instance, a doctor's office) or at a "facility" (such as a hospital).

[7] There have been three five-year reviews, reflected in the work expense RVUs for the 1997, 2002, and 2007 fee schedules. RVUs may also be changed because of annual refinements or budget-neutrality adjustments.

[8] The work expense RVUs have always been based on the resources that a physician uses to provide a service. In contrast, the practice expense and malpractice expense RVUs were initially based on historical charges and were switched to a resource-based methodology only in later years. The resource-based practice expense RVUs were phased in from 1999 to 2002, and the resource-based malpractice expense RVUs were instituted in 2000. By law, those changes had to be budget neutral: Total expenditures had to remain the same under the new resource-based method as they would have been according to the charge-based method. Consequently, budget neutrality implies that some services would receive higher payments while others would receive lower payments.

[9] Revisions to GPCIs are phased in over a two-year period if more than one year has passed since the last revision. There were revisions in 1995, 1998, 2001, 2004, and 2005. The Medicare Prescription Drug Improvement and Modernization Act of 2003, or MMA (P.L. 109-432), established a temporary floor of 1.0 for the work component GPCI from 2004 to 2006, as an additional means to increase payments to rural areas. The Tax Relief and Health Care Act of 2006 (P.L. 108-73) extends the GPCI floor for an additional year.

[10] This example utilizes service codes 99213 for an office visit and 62010 for treatment of a head injury. The carrier number and locality codes for Manhattan are 00803 and 01, respectively; Alabama uses carrier number 00510 and locality code 00.

[11] Those adjustments, applied by means of "modifiers," can be smaller or greater than one. For example, partial procedures are paid at a reduced rate, whereas procedures with complications are paid at a higher rate than the fee schedule amount.

[12] The data show that roughly 90 percent of the services have actual payment rates within $1 of the fee schedule payment rates. Apart from the adjustments already mentioned, data errors also result in differences between fee schedule and actual payment rates.

[13] Annual changes in payment rates for physicians' services are mainly the result of updates in the conversion factor. In some years, there have been additional reasons for changes in payment rates arising from revisions to RVUs and GPCIs, and from budget-neutrality adjustments.

[14] Per-beneficiary spending is calculated using actual payment rates or Medicare allowed charges, which include both Medicare's share of payments and that paid by beneficiaries through cost sharing (in the form of deductibles and copayments). See Table A-1 in the appendix for Medicare's total spending for physicians' services and the number of beneficiaries enrolled in the program between 1997 and 2005.

[15] Using the consumer price index to control for inflation, rather than the MEI, does not change the above figures (or any of the analysis in this paper) in a significant way.

[16] The comparison includes spending for hospital inpatient care, skilled nursing facilities, hospice care, and home health services under Part A, as well as spending for other professional and outpatient ancillary services, and services provided in other facilities, under Part B.

[17] A carrier is a private company that has a contract with Medicare to pay physicians and most other providers of Medicare Part B services. Carrier numbers and locality codes define geographic locations that determine, in part, Medicare payment rates for physicians' services through the use of GPCIs.

[18] Services included in the claims data but not covered under the fee schedule are excluded. Anesthesia services are also excluded because they are reimbursed under a separate fee schedule. In addition, ambulatory surgical

center claims and Railroad Retirement Board claims, neither of which is assigned to the physician payment localities, are excluded from the analysis.

[19] For observations with invalid carrier or locality codes, values are imputed using zip codes from a 2002 CMS zip code to carrier file.

[20] For clarity, the payment rate for a given service is referred to as price, or P, and volume and intensity are referred to as quantity, or Q. The rest of the paper refers to prices and payment rates interchangeably. Quantity and volume and intensity of physicians' services are used interchangeably as well.

[21] To calculate annual spending on physicians' services, payments made for all claims submitted in a given year are totaled. That is, rather than counting the number of services of each type and multiplying that number by an average price, each service is treated as unique in order to retain the variation in the different components of price. As previously mentioned, spending totals include Medicare's payments and beneficiaries' obligations in the form of deductibles and copayments.

[22] This decomposition can also be written as $P^{t+1} \cdot Q^{t+1} - P^t \cdot Q^t = P^t \cdot \Delta Q + \Delta P\, Q^{t+1}$. The main results of the paper remain unchanged when using the different reference period.

[23] In both terms, "counterfactual" spending is computed as per-beneficiary spending in year $t+1$ with physicians' services set at year t levels, or $P^{t+1} Q^t$. Note that, while the conversion factor and the RVUs for year $t+1$ are known, the adjustment factor in year $t+1$ is not. Therefore, for each physician service, the adjustment factor in year $t+1$ is estimated as the ratio of the sum of actual payments and the sum of fee schedule payment rates in year t.

[24] That adjustment had been put in place in 1997 for the purpose of offsetting increases in spending that arose from the five-year review of work expense RVUs.

[25] Because the analysis is done at the per-beneficiary level, the observed changes in spending cannot be attributed to changes in enrollment levels.

[26] See, for example, Kenneth E. Thorpe, "The Rise in Health Care Spending and What to Do About It," *Health Affairs*, vol. 24, no. 6 (November/December 2005), pp. 1436–1445; and Department of Health and Human Services, Centers for Medicare and Medicaid Services, *Review of Assumptions and Methods of the Medicare Trustees' Financial Projections* (prepared by the 2000 Technical Review Panel on Medicare Trustees Reports, December 2000), available at www.cms.hhs.gov/ ReportsTrustFunds/downloads/TechnicalPanel Report 2000.pdf.

[27] In order to assess the impact of demographic changes on spending, the sample is divided into 48 such categories: age (4), sex (2), race (3), and death (2). Then, predicted per-beneficiary spending in 2005 is computed holding the demographic composition as it was in 1997.

[28] Those figures are based on changes in the distribution of Medicare enrollees with positive spending. Replicating this analysis using changes in demographic characteristics of all Medicare enrollees yields similar results.

[29] Additionally, new and newly covered services can also have an impact on the volume of existing services. For example, the addition of preventative services to the Medicare fee schedule could lead to increases in office visits as well as any follow-up treatment, but it could also decrease some services as a result of the early detection of certain conditions or illnesses.

[30] See Kaiser Family Foundation, *Trends and Indicators in the Changing Health Care Marketplace*, "Section 2: Health Insurance Enrollment," Exhibit 2.17 (publication no. 7031, updated February 8, 2006), available at www.kff.org/insurance/7031/index.cfm.

[31] See Medicare Payment Advisory Commission, *Report to the Congress: Medicare Payment Policy*, "Section 2B: Physician Services" (March 2007), available at www.medpac.gov/publications/ congressional_reports/Mar07_EntireReport.pdf.

[32] Evidence from the RAND Health Insurance experiment supports the notion that patients respond to different cost-sharing schemes. For a summary of the results of the RAND experiment, see Joseph P. Newhouse, *Free for All? Lessons from the RAND Health Insurance Experiment* (Cambridge, Mass.: Harvard University Press, 1993). It should be noted, however, that a vast majority of fee-for-service Medicare beneficiaries have supplemental coverage. Thus, any behavioral response may be weakened, given that some beneficiaries are not responsible for the full change in payment rates.

[33] See Thomas G. McGuire and Mark V. Pauly, "Physician Response to Fee Changes with Multiple Payers," *Journal of Health Economics*, vol. 10 (1991), pp. 385–410.

[34] Measuring the behavioral response of physicians' services is not straightforward because those services are heterogeneous, ranging from a simple office visit to a complicated procedure. One solution to this problem has been to convert those services into RVUs, which provides a homogeneous measure of quantity. Similarly, converting Medicare fees into allowed Medicare payment per RVU provides a measure of price.

[35] See, for example, Jack Hadley and James D. Reschovsky, "Medicare Fees and Physicians' Medicare Service Volume: Beneficiaries Treated and Services per Beneficiary," *International Journal of Health Care Finance Economics*, vol. 6, issue 2 (2006), pp. 131–150.

[36] The empirical literature has not addressed the extent to which the observed relationship between changes in payment rates and changes in volume is the result of beneficiaries responding to fee changes. In addition,

because of data availability restrictions, the majority of the empirical research has not explicitly accounted for substitution across Medicare and private services.

[37] Nguyen Xuan Nguyen and Frederick William Derrick, "Physician Behavioral Response to a Medicare Price Reduction," *Health Services Research*, vol. 32, no. 3 (August 1997), pp. 283–298.

[38] See also Stephen Zuckerman, Stephen A. Norton, and Diana Verrilli, "Price Controls and Medicare Spending: Assessing the Volume Offset Assumption," *Medical Care Research and Review*, vol. 55, no. 4 (December 1998), pp. 457–483. The study estimates behavioral responses to fee changes over a seven-year period (1986 to 1992) across services and specialties. Pooling all service types, specialties, and years, the authors estimate a volume offset of 17 percent. The regressions for different service types suggest statistically significant volume offsets, ranging from -0.61 for procedures and -0.16 to -0.25 for tests and imaging. For evaluation and management services, whose fees increased on average during this period, the authors estimate a volume offset of -0.27. Other results are consistent with previous research in that behavioral responses are largest for surgical specialties and obstetrics (-0.54 to -0.75) and smaller for cardiology and urology (-0.32). No effects are seen in gastroenterology or ophthalmology. Unexpectedly, regression results for internal medicine suggest an elasticity of 0.24.

[39] Ibid.

[40] Centers for Medicare and Medicaid Services, "Physician Volume and Intensity Response," Office of the Actuary memorandum (August 13, 1998), available at www.cms.hhs.gov/ActuarialStudies/ downloads/PhysicianResponse.pdf. This study is based on Medicare claims data from 1994 to 1996.

[41] This analysis employs the same data as that used in the decomposition analysis presented earlier.

[42] In order to test the symmetry assumption, the model is modified so that spending in year $t+1$ is regressed on $(1 + G) \cdot P^{t+1} \cdot Q^t + D R_I \cdot (P^{t+1} \cdot Q^t - P^t \cdot Q^t) + (1 - D) \cdot R \cdot (P^{t+1} \cdot Q^t - P^t \cdot Q^t)$. In this specification, D equals 1 when payment rates fall between years t and $t+1$, and 0 otherwise; R_I and R_D are the coefficients for the estimates of the behavioral response when payment rates increase and decrease, respectively. The symmetry assumption is evaluated by a statistical comparison of the estimates for R_I and R_D.

[43] Given the possibility that the behavioral response may not be observed immediately, a different specification is also modeled, where the behavioral response is a function of changes in payment rates between years t and $t+1$ and years $t-1$ and t. In other words, predicted spending in year $t+1$ is given by: Predicted spending$^{t+1} = (1 + G) \cdot P^{t+1} \cdot Q^t + R \cdot (P^{t+1} \cdot Q^t - P^t \cdot Q^t) + R_{-1} \cdot (P^t \cdot Q^{t-1} - P^{t-1} \cdot Q^{t-1})$, where R is the behavioral response parameter between years t and $t+1$ and R_{-1} is the behavioral response parameter for changes in payment rates between years $t-1$ and t. Regression results for this specification do not support the hypothesis that a lagged response exists. The coefficient on R_{-1} equals 0.131 and is statistically insignificant. The rest of the coefficients remain quantitatively similar and of the same statistical significance as those shown in Table 5. That result may not be surprising because Medicare's physician fee schedule is available to physicians well in advance of the start of the year. Furthermore, to the extent that beneficiaries are less aware of the changes, this evidence may support the notion that the behavioral response estimated is driven by physicians and not by beneficiaries.

[44] In order to test whether the results are driven by years in which increases in spending were higher than in other years—1999 to 2001—Model 1 is run without these observations. Although such a test relies on only five years of aggregate data, the results are both quantitatively and qualitatively similar to those of the full sample.

[45] Also, that the behavioral responses could be opposite in sign is difficult to accept because that would imply the conclusion that Medicare payment rates for physicians' services happen to be at the level that minimizes the quantity of services.

[46] To the extent that private and Medicare fees are correlated, the omission of private fees in the estimated models could result in biased behavioral response estimates.

[47] As mentioned in the text, in terms of budgetary implications, the source of the behavioral response is irrelevant.

In: Medicare: A Primer
Editor: Alice R. Williamson

ISBN: 978-1-60741-108-6
© 2009 Nova Science Publishers, Inc.

Chapter 3

IMPROVING MEDICARE EFFICIENCY AND VALUE

Medicare Payment Advisory Commission
Subcommittee on Health Committee on Energy and Commerce
U.S. House of Representatives

Chairman Pallone, Ranking Member Deal, distinguished Subcommittee members, I am Mark Miller, Executive Director of the Medicare Payment Advisory Commission (MedPAC). I appreciate the opportunity to be here with you this morning to discuss MedPAC's perspectives on ways to bring greater efficiency to Medicare. MedPAC has sought improvements in Medicare efficiency above and beyond our legislative mandate over the last several years, evidenced in our ongoing work on payment adequacy for Medicare fee-for-service (FFS) payment systems and payments to managed care plans under the Medicare Advantage (MA) program, as well as specific work on pay-forperformance, coordination of care, bundling of medical services, comparative effectiveness, and a host of more targeted studies on specific elements of Medicare payment policy such as payments for imaging services and the sustainable growth rate under the Medicare physician fee schedule. I would like to discuss several of these areas in greater detail today.

There is currently a great deal of interest in improving the efficiency of the Medicare program. This interest is driven not only by the desire to make Medicare a better program but also by growing concern about the sustainability of Medicare spending. Medicare as a public payer has suffered from the same persistently high growth in health care cost that has plagued all sectors of the health financing community. Medicare spending grew 9.3 percent annually between 1980 and 2004, on average, considerably higher than the average annual rate of growth in gross domestic product (GDP) of 6.5 percent for that same period. While growth in GDP—the measure of goods and services produced in the United States—is used as a benchmark of how much additional growth in expenditure society can afford, other measures illustrate the more direct impacts of growth in Medicare spending on the program's beneficiaries. Between 1970 and 2005, the average monthly Social Security benefit increased by an inflation-adjusted average annual rate of 1.6 percent; during the same period, Medicare Supplementary Medical Insurance premiums grew by more than 4 percent annually. Recent

Part B premium increases have offset 30 percent to 40 percent of the dollar increase in the average Social Security benefit. Yet, despite this rapid growth in spending, a large body of evidence suggests the increased cost of health care has not come with a corresponding increase in quality. The Institute of Medicine, in its 2001 report *Crossing the Quality Chasm*, suggested that while care may be improving in many settings, significant gaps remain between what is known to be good care and the care delivered, and it is still all too common for beneficiaries not to receive high-quality health care.

Slowing the increase in Medicare outlays is important; indeed it is becoming urgent. Medicare's rising costs, particularly when coupled with the projected growth in the number of beneficiaries, threaten to place a significant burden on taxpayers. It is likely that all available tools (efficiency gains, efforts to combat fraud and abuse, tax increases, and benefit restructuring) will be necessary to address the financial pressures facing Medicare. Much of MedPAC's work focuses on improved efficiency—getting more in terms of quality and outcomes for each Medicare dollar spent—as a way to help address Medicare's growing financial crisis.

The Commission has implicitly or explicitly dealt with the role of efficiency in many aspects of its ongoing work:

- *Payment updates.* Ensuring that provider productivity is taken into account in estimating recommended payment updates for FFS providers and identifying situations when payments are more than adequate;

- *Payment accuracy.* Ensuring that payments for health care goods and services accurately reflect providers' costs so that adverse incentives are not created (e.g., to select patients and provide higher profit services in lieu of services that provide the best outcomes);

- *Bundling.* Creating larger units of payment to give providers flexibility in the efficient provision of care, while minimizing incentives to increase profits by providing additional services;

- *MA plans.* Ensuring that capitated rates paid to plans are neutral to Medicare FFS, so plans have the incentive to be efficient, and so that beneficiaries will be able to make choices about their coverage options based on "apples to apples" comparisons;

- *Pay-for-performance programs.* Designing payment system incentives to provide high-quality, appropriate care;

- *Measuring provider resource use.* Using Medicare administrative data to let providers know how their service utilization compares with that of their peers;

- *Care coordination.* Increasing quality of care and decreasing costs when multiple providers are involved by implementing payment incentives that promote coordination and thus reduce adverse advents such as avoidable rehospitalizations following discharge; and

- *Comparative effectiveness.* Ensuring that new health care treatments and technologies represent advances in quality or efficiency in making health care decisions.

MedPAC believes there is considerable opportunity for improvements in program efficiency to increase the incentives for more efficient delivery of health care and, in so doing, help constrain the growth of program spending and increase the value of each dollar spent. Pricing policies can be powerful tools in creating these incentives; other program policies can complement changes to the payment systems. The likelihood of success of these measures in controlling spending will be enhanced if Medicare and other public programs can collaborate with private sector payers to ensure that these incentives' are put in place across the board, rather than only in Medicare.

MedPAC believes it is essential to look hard at the value of the services Medicare pays for. For three-quarters of the program's existence, Medicare's reimbursement for services was relatively indifferent to the quality of care provided. In general, as long as claims were submitted in accordance with applicable administrative and policy requirements, Medicare paid them, regardless of whether the quality of the service (to the extent it was even a consideration) was in the top 10 percent or the bottom 10 percent, regardless of whether it resulted in an improved outcome for the patient, and regardless of whether the service was the most appropriate for a given patient with a given condition. Persistent growth in Medicare spending led to passage of the watershed Balanced Budget Act of 1997 (BBA), which implemented a number of significant reforms to the program, most notably new prospective payment systems for providers that had previously been reimbursed on the basis of their costs and a new managed care program, Medicare+Choice. The rationale for the Medicare+Choice program was driven, at least in part, by the notion that managed care plans could deliver care to Medicare beneficiaries more efficiently than traditional FFS and thus in the long run would provide greater value for both the program and its beneficiaries. Such efficiencies would be leveraged even further by competition among plans, and one of the dimensions upon which plans were explicitly expected to compete was quality. Quality was also invoked in the BBA's authorization of a number of demonstration projects on the competitive acquisition of certain durable medical equipment.

The quality of care beneficiaries receive is not assured. Evidence shows that beneficiaries do not always receive the care they need and too often the care they do get is not high quality. There are also significant geographic variations in the amount of services beneficiaries receive, with little or no relationship to outcomes. This variation in care may expose some beneficiaries to unnecessary risk and is costly to beneficiaries and to the program.

Given the financial pressures facing Medicare, the program can no longer be indifferent to the value of the health care it pays for on behalf of its beneficiaries. The program must focus not only on achieving efficiency through calibrating payments, it must also pay much more attention to the quality and outcomes of the care its beneficiaries receive—in essence, looking not only at the price of health care but also at the value of the care that is purchased for that price.

PAYMENT UPDATES

Each year, the Commission recommends payment updates and other policy changes for FFS Medicare. To help determine the appropriate level of aggregate funding for a given payment system, the Commission considers whether current Medicare payments are adequate by examining information about beneficiaries' access to care; changes in provider supply and capacity; volume and quality of care; providers' access to capital; and, where available, the relationship of Medicare payments to providers' costs. As mandated by the Congress, MedPAC explicitly considers efficiency in making these assessments: Ideally, Medicare's payments should not exceed the costs of the efficient providers. Efficient providers use fewer inputs to produce quality services. We then account for expected cost changes in the next payment year, such as those resulting from changes in input prices.

Improvements in productivity should reduce providers' costs in the coming year. Medicare's payment systems should encourage providers to reduce the quantity of inputs required to produce a unit of service by at least a modest amount each year while maintaining service quality. Thus, in most cases where payments are adequate, some amount representing productivity improvement should be subtracted from the initial update value, which is usually an estimate of the change in input prices. Consequently, we apply a policy goal for improvement in productivity. This factor links Medicare's expectations for efficiency to the gains achieved by the firms and workers who pay taxes that fund Medicare. Under this construct, MedPAC has identified instances in which payments are more than adequate and, on several occasions in recent years, has recommended no annual updates to provider payments. Most recently, in our March 2007 report to the Congress, we produced a number of update recommendations for the 2008 payment year cognizant of potential provider efficiency gains that will generate program savings if implemented:

- Skilled nursing facility (SNF) services. The Commission recommended that the Congress eliminate the update to payment rates for SNF services for fiscal year 2008;
- Home health services. The Commission recommended that the Congress eliminate the update to payment rates for home health care services for calendar year 2008;
- Inpatient rehabilitation facility (IRF) services. The Commission recommended that the Congress update payment rates for IRFs for fiscal year 2008 by 1 percent;
- Long-term care hospitals (LTCH). MedPAC recommended that the Secretary eliminate the update to payment rates for LTCH services for 2008.

Medicare should exert continued financial pressure on providers to control their costs, much as would happen in a competitive marketplace. We have found, for example, that hospitals under financial pressure tend to control cost growth better than those that have non-Medicare revenues that greatly exceed their costs. The Commission is striving to pursue innovative means to increase value in Medicare while maintaining financial pressure in all its payment systems to restrain costs.

PAYMENT ACCURACY

Another component of encouraging efficiency through payment policy is to ensure that Medicare's payments for health care services are accurate. Misvalued services can distort the price signals for a wide variety of health care services. Some overvalued services may be overprovided because they are more profitable than others. Under Medicare Part B, mispricing may exacerbate the volume-inducing effects of the physician fee schedule. We identified similar situations in Part A. For example, our 2005 analysis of specialty hospitals showed that certain kinds of physician-owned specialty hospitals were extremely adept at identifying (and focusing on) more profitable diagnosis related groups (DRGs), and within those DRGs, the least sick (and most profitable) patients. By contrast, undervalued services may prompt providers to increase volume to maintain their overall level of payment. Conversely, some providers may opt not to furnish undervalued services, which can threaten access to care. For example, MedPAC has identified potential problems with Medicare's payment systems for both SNFs and hospices that may underpay and thus discourage these providers from accepting Medicare patients with complex medical conditions requiring expensive drug or nontherapy ancillary regimens as part of their treatment.

A service can become overvalued for a number of reasons. For example, under Medicare's physician fee schedule, the amount of physician work needed to furnish a service may decline as physicians become more proficient or when new technologies are incorporated. Services can also become overvalued when practice expenses decline. Likewise, services can become undervalued when physician work increases or practice expenses rise. Although CMS reviews the relative values assigned to physician services every 5 years, some services likely continue to be misvalued. In recent years, per capita volume for different types of services has grown at widely disparate rates, with volume growth in imaging and minor procedures outpacing that for visits and major procedures. Volume growth differs across services for several reasons, including variability in the extent to which demand for services can be induced and advances in technology that expand access and can improve patient outcomes. The Commission and others have voiced concerns, however, that differential growth in volume is due in part to differences in the profitability of services.

Differences in the profitability of services send signals to the market that go beyond incentives to over- or underfurnish services. For example, certain types of overvalued physician services may become more concentrated in some specialties than in others, such as primary care, that provide proportionately more low-profit services (such as evaluation and management services) that are less amenable to productivity gains. Facing these incentives, new physicians may be less willing to choose specialties that frequently provide undervalued services, resulting in reduced beneficiary access to certain physicians and certain services.

MedPAC has analyzed the issue of payment accuracy at great length in the context of Medicare's physician payment system. The Commission concluded in its March 2006 report to the Congress that CMS's process for reviewing the work relative values of physician services must be improved. To maintain the integrity of the physician fee schedule, we recommended that CMS play a lead role in identifying overvalued services so that they are not ignored in the process of revising the fee schedule's relative weights. We also recommended that CMS establish a group of experts, separate from the Relative Value Scale Update Committee (RUC), to help the agency conduct these and other activities. This recommendation was intended not to supplant the RUC but to augment it. To that end, the group should include members who do not directly benefit from changes to Medicare's payment rates, such as experts in medical economics and technology diffusion and physicians who are employed by managed care organizations and academic medical centers. The Commission also urged CMS to update the data and assumptions it uses to estimate the practice expenses associated with physician services.

Ensuring the accuracy of payments to other providers—including hospitals and post-acute care providers—is also important. To this end, the Commission recommended refinements to the DRGs used in Medicare's hospital inpatient prospective payment system to capture differences in severity of illness among patients and thus reduce the potential for differential profitability of DRGs or individual patients within DRGs. We also recommended improving the case-mix systems used in Medicare's payment systems for post-acute care services, most notably the payment groups used under the SNF prospective payment system (PPS), to provide appropriate incentives for SNFs to treat patients requiring nontherapy ancillary services.

We recognize that CMS has many priorities and limited resources and that refinements to the various payment systems to ensure accuracy of payments will raise some difficult technical issues. These include the potentially increasing the number of payment groups, possible increases in spending from improvements in coding, and others. The Congress should take steps to ensure that CMS has the resources it needs to make the recommended refinements to Medicare's payment systems.

BUNDLING

Another way to promote efficiency through pricing in the delivery of health care services to Medicare beneficiaries is through "bundling." In bundling, a single payment is made for a group of related services, rather than making individual payments for each service in the group. A larger unit of payment puts physicians and other providers at greater financial risk for the services provided and thus gives them an incentive to provide and order services judiciously. Medicare already bundles preoperative and follow-up physician visits into global payments for surgical services. Candidates for further bundling include services typically provided during the same episode of care, particularly those episodes for conditions with clear guidelines but large variations in actual use of service, such as diabetes treatment. In identifying the best candidates for bundling, one must consider that, while bundled payments could lead to fewer unnecessary services, they could also lead to stinting or unbundling (e.g., referring patients to other providers for services that should be included in a bundle). Medicare should explore options for increasing the size of the unit of payment to include bundles of services that physicians often furnish together or during the same episode of care, similar to the approach used in the hospital inpatient PPS.

MedPAC will be examining bundling the hospital payment and physician payment for a given DRG and for groups of DRGs, which could increase efficiency and improve coordination of care. This approach to bundling could be expanded in the future to capture periods of time (e.g., 1 or 2 weeks) after the admission but likely to include care (e.g., post-acute care, physician services) strongly related to the admission, further boosting efficiency and coordination across sites of care. We have also recommended broader bundling of services for patients with end-stage renal disease, most notably suggesting the inclusion of erythropoietin in the payment bundle (see above) to reduce the incentive to provide more of a given item or service to reap greater profits. Bundling services could be structured so that savings go to the providers, the program, or both.

MEDICARE ADVANTAGE

The Commission has discussed the concept of efficiency at great length with respect to the MA program. Many of the positions and principles the Commission has adopted with respect to increasing efficiency through pricing of individual services or groups of services also apply to the calculation of payments for even larger groups of services—to wit, the capitated payments paid to managed care plans under MA. The Commission has always supported a private plan option in Medicare, given the potential savings and expanded beneficiary choice the private plans can bring to Medicare.

In our March report, the Commission presented recent findings on the MA plans beneficiaries can join in lieu of traditional FFS Medicare. While the initial intent of the MA program may have been predicated on the idea that managed care represented a less costly alternative to FFS Medicare, our most recent findings suggest that payments to plans are generally higher—in some cases much higher—than corresponding payments would have been on behalf of the same beneficiaries under traditional FFS. The Commission believes that greater efficiency is achieved when organizations face financial pressure. The Medicare program needs to exert consistent financial pressure on both the traditional FFS program and the MA program. This financial pressure, coupled with meaningful measurement of quality and resource use to reward efficient care, will maximize the value of Medicare for the taxpayers and beneficiaries who finance the program.

Table 1. Medicare Advantage benchmarks and payments in 2006 exceed expected Medicare fee-for-service expenditures for all types of plans

	HMO/POS/PSO*	Local PPOs*	Regional PPO*	PFFS
Enrollment as of July 2006 (in thousands)	5,195	285	82	774
Enrollment as of February 2007 (in thousands)	5,063	333	109	1,328
Net enrollment growth	-3%	17%	33%	72%
Benchmark relative to FFS cost	115%	120	112	122
Payments relative to FFS cost	110%	117	110	119
Bid (for Medicare A/B benefit) relative to FFS	97%	108%	103%	109%

Note: POS (provider of service), PSO (provider-sponsored organization), PPO (preferred provider organization), PFFS (private fee-for-service), FFS (fee-for-service). Payments relative to expected FFS costs for the beneficiaries enrolled in Medicare Advantage plans.

  * Data exclude special needs plans.

Source: MedPAC analysis of data from CMS on plan bids, enrollment, and benchmarks.

Medicare's private plan option was originally designed as a program that would produce efficiency in the delivery of health care. Efficient plans could be able to provide extra benefits to enrollees choosing to enroll in such plans, and better efficiency would lead to higher plan enrollment. Unfortunately, MA has instead become a program with few incentives for efficiency. Although MA uses "bidding" as the means of determining plan payments and beneficiary premiums, the bids are against benchmarks that are not competitively set. Setting benchmarks well above the cost of traditional Medicare signals that the program welcomes plans that are more costly than traditional Medicare. Inefficient plans—as well as efficient plans—are able to provide the kind of enhanced coverage that attracts beneficiaries to private plans because of generous MA program payments that are in excess of Medicare FFS payment levels. All taxpayers, and all Medicare beneficiaries—not just the 18 percent of beneficiaries enrolled in private plans—are funding the payments in excess of Medicare FFS levels.

Our analysis of MA payments shows that the benchmarks (which are the reference level for plan bids and the maximum program payment) now average 116 percent of traditional Medicare FFS levels, and payments average 112 percent. The ratio of benchmarks and payments varies by plan type, although it exceeds the expected Medicare FFS expenditures for those beneficiaries for all types of plans. Table 1 shows that payments to HMOs are 110 percent of expected FFS costs. Payments for private FFS (PFFS) plans are 119 percent of expected Medicare FFS costs, because they are located in areas of the country where benchmarks are much greater than FFS, and because they are relatively inefficient at returning benefits to their enrollees.

Private plans are given the flexibility and the incentives to improve the delivery of care and bargain with providers to negotiate payment rates that are expected to create program savings. However, the excess payments to private plans allow them to be less efficient than they would otherwise have to be, because inefficient plans can use the excess payments— rather than savings from efficiencies—to finance extra benefits that in turn attract enrollees to such plans. As shown in Table 1, enrollment has grown substantially in MA as result of this situation. In 2006, 17 percent of beneficiaries were enrolled in MA plans, a level close to its all-time high.

Strikingly, almost half the growth in 2006 was in PFFS MA plans—the highest-paid and thus arguably least efficient—of the available types of MA plans. PFFS plans are nearly identical to Medicare FFS but with an added layer of marketing, operating and administrative costs, and profits. If the growth in enrollment in these plans reflected beneficiary preferences in the form of their willingness to pay higher premiums, such patterns would reflect a perceived benefit. However, it is likely that this growth has been fueled by program subsidies. PFFS plans primarily draw their enrollment from higher benchmark counties—specifically counties that were historically "floor" counties. MA benchmarks in these counties reflect a minimum payment level established by statute, resulting in benchmarks far above FFS expenditure levels in most cases. The statutory floor thus provides an implicit subsidy for these plans, and thus it is difficult to see the additional value such plans provide to Medicare beneficiaries for the additional cost to the program.

The Commission has always supported a private plan option in Medicare and has recommended lowering the MA benchmarks to help achieve a policy of financial neutrality between private plans and traditional Medicare FFS for several years. In addition to financial neutrality between MA and FFS, the Commission has also recommended neutrality between types of MA plans, including eliminating the stabilization fund for preferred provider organization plans and making bidding rules consistent across plan types. Further, the Commission has recommended a pay-forperformance program for MA plans, and calculating clinical measures for the FFS program that would permit CMS to compare quality in the FFS program with that in MA plans.

OBTAINING GREATER VALUE

Ideally, payment systems not only reflect efficient and accurate pricing, but also give providers incentives to furnish better quality of care, to coordinate care (across settings, in chronic conditions), and to use resources judiciously. However, Medicare pays its providers the same regardless of the quality of their care, which perpetuates poor care for some beneficiaries, misspends program resources, and is unfair to high-performing providers. Medicare's payment system does not reward providers for coordinating patients' care across health care settings and providers, nor does it encourage the provision of preventive and primary care services, even though such actions may improve quality of care and reduce costs.

To change payment incentives, the Congress and CMS must adopt policies that link payment to the quality of care provided. MedPAC's pay-for-performance recommendations would go some way toward correcting the problem of lack of incentives for quality care. At the same time, Medicare needs to explore measuring provider resource use and to encourage coordination of care and provision of primary care.

COMPARATIVE EFFECTIVENESS

Increasing the value of the Medicare program to beneficiaries and taxpayers requires knowledge about the costs and health outcomes of services. Until more information on the comparative effectiveness of new and existing health care treatments and technologies is available, patients, providers, and the program will have difficulty determining what constitutes good-quality care and effective use of resources.

Comparative-effectiveness information, which compares the outcomes associated with different therapies for the same condition, could help Medicare use its resources more efficiently. Comparative effectiveness has the potential to identify medical services that are more likely to improve patient outcomes and discourage the use of services with fewer benefits. CMS already assesses the clinical effectiveness of services when making decisions about national coverage and paying for some services, but to date FFS Medicare has not routinely used comparative information on the costs of services. Medicare Part D plans and other payers and providers, however, such as the Veterans Health Administration, do use such information—for example, in drug formulary decision-making processes. Such information is critical for these entities, given the force of new technology in driving increased health care costs and the need for these payers to closely evaluate the comparative benefits of costly new technologies relative to existing treatments.

Private health plans and providers have not been at the forefront of effectiveness research. Private payers and providers may be reluctant to use comparative-effectiveness information extensively for fear that patients will criticize them as being more concerned about cutting costs than about patients' health. Litigation risks may also dissuade some private payers from using comparative-effectiveness information. In addition, private payers may anticipate problems keeping the information proprietary (thus aiding their competitors) and may fear that it would be difficult to capture the full return on their investment.

Medicare could use comparative-effectiveness information in a number of ways to improve the value of care beneficiaries receive. Medicare could use such information to inform providers and patients about the value of services, since there is some evidence developed by the Sacramento Healthcare Decisions group in 2001 and by Marjorie Ginsburg in 2004 that both might consider comparative-effectiveness information when weighing treatment options. Medicare might also use the information to prioritize pay-for-performance measures, target screening programs, or prioritize disease management initiatives. In addition, Medicare could use comparative-effectiveness information in its rate-setting process.

Given the potential utility of comparative-effectiveness information to the Medicare program, an increased role of the federal government in sponsoring the research may be warranted. Concerns have been raised by Moher and colleagues in the *Annals of Internal Medicine* about the variability and lack of transparency in methods and by Bekelman and colleagues regarding the potential bias of industry-sponsored researchers conducting clinical- and cost-effectiveness research. MedPAC inventoried many of these concerns in our June 2006 report to the Congress.

A public-private partnership may more effectively address stakeholders' concerns about the use of comparative-effectiveness analysis than a noncollaborative process. A partnership that defines analytic standards would send researchers a clear, effective signal to improve their methods and develop valid and transparent comparative-effectiveness analyses. A partnership could help set priorities for clinical-effectiveness review and research. Services could be selected based on disease prevalence, high per unit cost, high total expenditures, and other factors.

Implementing the findings from comparative-effectiveness analysis may not save money for the Medicare program. Wider use of cost-effective, underutilized services could result in increased Medicare spending, which might not be offset with savings elsewhere. On the other hand, over the long run, comparative-effectiveness research could save the Medicare program money if it encourages manufacturers to develop services that are more cost-effective than current ones or if it helps inform providers and influences their patterns of care.

PAY-FOR-PERFORMANCE PROGRAMS

Medicare has a responsibility to ensure that its beneficiaries have access to high-quality care. Yet beneficiaries receive care from a system known to have problems with quality. Beth McGlynn and fellow researchers have noted that care is improving in many settings, but significant gaps remain between what is known to be good care and the care delivered. For example, Cathy Schoen, Karen Davis, and coauthors reported in 2006 that only about half the adults in the United States receive all recommended clinical screening tests and preventive services, and many quality indicators vary widely across states.

Measures of quality and guidelines for appropriate care are increasingly available. The Medicare program has been a leading force in efforts to develop and use quality measures, often leading initiatives to publicly disclose quality information, standardize tools for data collection, and give feedback to providers for improvement. CMS has also revised its regulatory standards to require that providers, such as hospitals and home health agencies, have quality improvement systems in place. CMS is conducting a number of demonstrations to explore whether financial incentives can improve the quality of care providers furnish. CMS's focus on quality provides a strong foundation for future initiatives.

While these tools can begin to improve quality, financial disincentives to improve quality allow the quality gap to persist. Medicare pays all health care providers without differentiating on the basis of quality. Those providers who improve quality are not rewarded for their efforts. In fact, Medicare often pays more when poor care results in complications that require additional treatment. The same negative or neutral incentives toward quality exist in the private sector. Many private purchasers and plans are experimenting with mechanisms to counterbalance these forces and reward those who provide high-quality care. Yet, they agree that Medicare's participation in these efforts is critical because of its market power and because private sector efforts alone may take a much longer time to show effects.

In a series of reports, we have recommended that Medicare change the incentives of the system by basing a portion of provider payment on performance. In our June 2003 report to the Congress, we established criteria for measures to compare providers to determine whether pay for performance is feasible in settings where Medicare beneficiaries receive care. The Commission also developed design principles to provide guidance on how to administer and fund a pay-for-performance program, which should:

- Reward providers based on improving care and exceeding certain benchmarks,
- Be funded by initially setting aside a small proportion of payments,
- Distribute all payments that are set aside to providers who achieve the quality criteria, and
- Establish a process through which measures can continue to evolve.

In our March 2004 report to the Congress, we found that MA plans and the facilities and physicians that care for dialysis patients were settings where pay-for-performance strategies could be implemented. In our March 2005 report to the Congress, we evaluated the available measures and measurement activities for physicians by our criteria and found useful structural, process, and patient experience indicators. Outcomes measures could be used with additional data and research. Therefore, we recommended that the Congress establish a quality incentive payment policy for physicians in Medicare. We also recommended pay-for-performance strategies for hospitals and home health agencies. While such efforts are important in increasing the quality of care provided to Medicare beneficiaries, it is important to note that MedPAC does not consider adjusting payments to reflect quality of care to be the end goal of pay-for-performance systems. Rather, we believe that once the link between payments and quality is well established, Medicare should then use the "payment" aspect of pay for performance to further drive increased efficiency—reflected by the combination of quality and cost—in delivering health care service.

MEASURING PROVIDER RESOURCE USE

In addition to implementing incentives via payment systems through pay-forperformance type mechanisms, Medicare could use other means of getting providers to think more consciously about the services they provide and thus enlist them as more active partners in the effort to ensure efficient care. One way to do this, as MedPAC has recommended previously, would be for the program to consolidate data on provision of services at the level of individual providers. Medicare could identify physicians and other providers with very high resource use relative to their peers. CMS could initially provide confidential feedback to these providers on an informational basis only. Once greater experience and confidence in resource-use measurement tools were gained, policymakers could use the results for additional interventions such as public reporting, targeting fraud and abuse, pay for performance, or differential updates based on relative performance.

Measuring provider resource use relative to a peer group, and providing such information to the providers, would promote individual accountability and would enable providers to more readily see a link between their actions and Medicare spending overall. However, a number of technical issues would need to be resolved. Providers will need to be confident that their scores reflect the relative complexity of their patient mix and that they are being compared with an appropriate set of peers. There would likely be considerable controversy around initial scores as some providers realized that their practice patterns were not in line with those of their peers.

Table 2. Selected Boston cardiologist has higher clinical resource measurement for hypertension than his peers

	Overall patient complexity level (low to high)					
	All episodes	1	2	3	4	5
Stage 1 hypertension						
Number of episodes	141	41	45	35	13	7
Clinical resource use	$623	$453	$660	$814	$630	$410
Selected Boston cardiologist						
Average for all Boston cardiologists	$357	$251	$307	$369	$409	$450
Selected cardiologist's resource use score	*1.74*	*1.80*	*2.15*	*2.21*	*1.54*	*0.91*

Note: Stage indicates progression of the disease, with 1 being the mildest form. Overall complexity level indicates the presence of other diseases. Resource use score is the ratio of the cardiologist's resource use to the average for cardiologists in Boston.

Source: MedPAC analysis of 100 percent sample of 2001–2003 Medicare claims using the Medstat Episode Group grouper from Thomson Medstat.

MedPAC has made considerable progress in simulating how such a system might work in practice. In Table 2, we provide an example of comparing the resource use of an actual physician with the averages for his specialty within the market area. We demonstrate how the comparison can be broken down by type of case—both the stage of disease and the presence of comorbidities in patients. We then break down the comparison by the types of services that went into the selected episodes. The result is a comparison that can provide useful feedback to physicians about why their performance differs from that of their peers.

We use an individual cardiologist in Boston to compare a physician's clinical resource use with an overall expected value (an average across all specialties for the Boston metropolitan statistical area (MSA)) and with a specialty-specific expected value. We compare his actual clinical resource measurement with expected clinical resource measurement (based on the averages for all cardiologists treating hypertension in the Boston MSA) and calculate corresponding ratios. Ratios greater than 1.0 indicate higher than average values for clinical resource measurement (observed greater than expected) and ratios less than 1.0 indicate lower than average values for clinical resource measurement (observed lower than expected). When we use an expected clinical resource measurement value for cardiologists in Boston, his overall observed-to-expected ratio is 1.74, or not quite twice the average clinical resource measurement value.

MedPAC believes there is tremendous potential in making these comparisons of resource use and has recommended that Medicare collect and consolidate information on provider resource use and provide feedback on resource use to individual providers. Physicians would then be able to assess their practice styles, evaluate whether they tend to use more resources than their peers (or what available evidence-based research recommends), and revise their practice styles as appropriate. Once greater confidence with the measurement tool was gained, Medicare could use the results for payments—for example, as a component of a pay-for-performance program that rewards both quality and efficiency. CMS could also use the measurement tool to flag unusual patterns of care that might indicate misuse, fraud, and abuse.

CARE COORDINATION

In recent years, the Commission has explored multiple strategies to provide incentives for high-quality, low-cost care and thus improve efficiency in the Medicare program. However, even if individual providers are efficient, a beneficiary may still receive less-than-optimal care if providers do not communicate well with each other or if they do not monitor patient progress over time. To address this problem, we have considered ways to introduce care coordination and care management by creating incentives for providers to share clinical information with other providers, monitor patient status between visits, and fully communicate with patients about self-care.

The patients most in need of care coordination are those with multiple chronic conditions and other complex needs. Beneficiaries with chronic conditions represent a significant proportion of Medicare spending. In 2005, the Congressional Budget Office estimated that beneficiaries with more than one chronic condition made up 48 percent of the highest cost beneficiaries in 2001 but only 12 percent of the lowest cost beneficiary population. Yet, evidence continues to mount that beneficiaries with chronic conditions do not receive recommended care and may have hospitalizations that could have been avoided with better primary care. Researchers attribute this problem to poor monitoring of treatment— especially between visits—for beneficiaries and to a general lack of communication among providers. Coordinated care may improve patients' understanding of their conditions and compliance with medical advice and, in turn, reduce the use of high-cost settings such as emergency rooms and inpatient care. Ideally, care coordination will improve communication among providers, eliminating redundancy and improving quality.

Care coordination is difficult to accomplish in the FFS program because it requires managing patients across settings and over time, neither of which is supported by current payment methods or organizational structures. Further, because patients have the freedom to go to any willing physician or other provider, it is difficult to identify the practitioner most responsible for the patient's care, especially if the patient chooses to see multiple providers. The challenge is to find ways to create incentives in the FFS system to better coordinate care.

In our June 2006 report to the Congress, we outlined two illustrative care coordination models for complex patients in the FFS program: (1) Medicare could contract with providers in large or small groups that are capable of integrating the information technology and care manager infrastructure into patient clinical care, and (2) CMS could also contract with stand-alone care management organizations that would work with individual physicians. In either model, payment for services to coordinate care would be contingent on negotiated levels of performance in cost savings and quality improvements. Given that Medicare faces long-term sustainability problems and needs to learn more about the most cost-effective interventions, the entities furnishing the care managers and information systems should initially be required to produce some savings as a condition of payment. Demonstrating continued savings may not be necessary or feasible once strategies for coordinating care are broadly used.

MedPAC has illustrated one of the ways in which lack of care coordination is manifested by low-quality, high-cost care in its recent discussion of hospital readmissions from a post-acute care setting. Under the inpatient hospital PPS, hospitals have a strong incentive to reduce their costs, which can be achieved in part by reducing patient length of stay. They have little, if any, financial incentive to invest in managing post-hospital discharge transitions. In some cases, hospitals may discharge patients prematurely, resulting in a readmission to the hospital in the event that the patient's condition deteriorates at home or in a post-acute care setting as a result of the premature discharge. Readmissions may also occur as a result of discharges hobbled by incomplete coordination with a post-acute care provider. In such events, not only does the beneficiary receive lower quality (and potentially even life-threatening) care, but additional costs are added to Medicare. The Commission is exploring a two-step means of reducing readmission rates, first by publicly reporting hospital-specific readmission rates for a subset of conditions, followed by an adjustment to the underlying payment method to penalize hospitals with higher readmission rates.

Conclusion

In addition to taking efficiency into account when calculating payment rates or assessing the amount of annual provider payment updates, Medicare should institute policies that improve the value of the program to beneficiaries and taxpayers. Those policies should reward providers and health plans for efficient use of resources and create incentives to increase quality and coordinate care. Policies such as pay for performance that link payment to the quality of care physicians and other providers furnish should be implemented. At the same time, Medicare should encourage coordination of care and provision of primary care, bundle and package services where appropriate to reduce overuse, and ensure that its prices are accurate. To reduce unwarranted variation in volume and expenditures, Medicare should collect and distribute information about how providers' practice styles and use of resources compare with those of their peers. Ultimately, this information could be used to adjust payments to physicians. Findings from comparative-effectiveness research should be used to inform payment policy and furnished to beneficiaries and providers to inform decisions about medical care. Finally, concerted efforts should be made to identify and prevent misuse, fraud, and abuse by strengthening provider standards, ensuring that services are furnished by qualified providers to eligible recipients, and verifying that services are appropriate and billed accurately and that payments for those services are correct.

Because there are numerous payers in the U.S. health care system, achieving gains in efficiency is difficult for any one payer. To engender broader changes among providers, Medicare will likely need to collaborate with other payers but can take a leading role in driving change. But if we want Medicare to function more efficiently, the Congress needs to provide CMS with the necessary time, financial resources, and administrative flexibility. CMS will need to invest in information systems; develop, update, and improve measures of quality and resource use; and contract for specialized services. In the long run, failure to invest in CMS will result in higher program costs and lower quality of care.

In: Medicare: A Primer
Editor: Alice R. Williamson

ISBN: 978-1-60741-108-6
© 2009 Nova Science Publishers, Inc.

Chapter 4

MEDICARE: A PRIMER

Jennifer O'Sullivan

SUMMARY

Medicare is the nation's health insurance program for persons aged 65 and over and certain disabled persons. In FY2008, the program will cover an estimated 44.6 million persons (37.4 million aged and 7.3 million disabled) at a total cost of $459.4 billion. Federal costs (after deduction of beneficiary premiums and other offsetting receipts) will total $389.9 billion. In FY2008, federal Medicare spending will represent approximately 13% of the total federal budget and 3% of GDP. Medicare is an entitlement program, which means that it is required to pay for services provided to eligible persons, so long as specific criteria are met.

Since Medicare was enacted in 1965, it has undergone considerable changes. First, program coverage was expanded to include the disabled and persons with endstage renal disease (ESRD). Over time, increasing attention was placed on stemming the rapid increase in program spending, which outpaced projections, even in the initial years. This was typically achieved through tightening rules governing payments to providers of services and stemming the annual updates in such payments. The program moved from payments based on "reasonable costs" and "reasonable charges" to payment systems under which a pre-determined payment amount is established for a specified unit of service. At the same time, beneficiaries were given the option to obtain covered services through private managed care arrangements. Most Medicare payment provisions were incorporated into larger budget reconciliation bills designed to control overall federal spending.

In 2003, Congress enacted a major Medicare bill, the Medicare Prescription Drug, Improvement, and Modernization Act of 2003 (MMA). This legislation placed increasing emphasis on private sector management of benefits. It also created a new voluntary outpatient prescription drug benefit to be administered by private entities. Further, it introduced the concept of means testing into what had previously been strictly a social insurance program.

Congress continues to register concern about the rapid rise in Medicare spending and the ability of existing funding mechanisms to support the program over the longterm. A combination of factors has contributed to the rapid increase in Medicare costs. These include increases in overall medical costs, advances in health care delivery and medical technology, the aging of the population, and longer life spans. The issues confronting the program are not new; nor are the possible solutions likely to get any easier. For a number of years, various options have been suggested; however, legislative changes have focused on short-term issues. There is no consensus on the long-term approach that should be taken.

This report provides an overview of Medicare. It begins with a brief program history, and then outlines the key features of Parts A and B, also known as "Original Medicare." That is followed by overviews of Part C and Part D, a discussion of program financing, and a brief discussion of future program directions. It will be updated to reflect any legislative changes.

INTRODUCTION

Medicare is the nation's health insurance program for persons aged 65 and over and certain disabled persons. In FY2008, the program will cover an estimated 44.6 million persons (37.4 million aged and 7.3 million disabled)[1] at a total cost of $459.4 billion. Federal costs (after deduction of beneficiary premiums and other offsetting receipts) will total $389.9 billion.[2] In FY2008, federal Medicare spending will represent approximately 13% of the total federal budget and 3% of GDP.[3] Medicare is an entitlement program, which means that it is required to pay for services provided to eligible persons, so long as specific criteria are met. Spending under the program (except for a portion of administrative costs) is considered mandatory spending (not discretionary spending which is subject to the appropriations process).

Medicare serves approximately one in seven Americans and virtually all of the population aged 65 and over. In 2006 (the first year of the new drug benefit), Medicare spending accounted for an estimated 57% of federal health spending and 19% of all national health expenditures. Program spending represented 29% of national spending on hospital services, 21% of such spending for physicians and clinical services, and 18% of total drug spending (compared to 2% in 2005). In 2017, program spending is expected to account for 58% of federal spending and 21% of all national health expenditures. Spending in that year is expected to account for 31% of national spending on hospital services, 20% of such spending for physicians and clinical services, and 24% of total drug spending.[4]

The Medicare program is generally viewed as achieving its goal of helping aged and disabled persons meet many of their health care needs. However, the cost of the program and the significant year-to-year increases in such costs are a major concern for the Congress and other observers. The Congressional Budget Office (CBO) projects that program spending will double over the next ten years. The rapid growth rate reflects a number of factors, including overall increases in medical care costs (which typically exceed the rate of inflation in the economy as a whole), advances in health care delivery and medical technology, and longer life expectancies. Additional pressures will be placed on the program beginning in 2011, when baby boomers (persons born between 1946 and 1964) begin turning 65, the age when they become Medicare-eligible. For a number of years, Congress has looked at ways to stem the rapid increases in Medicare spending. This effort is likely to intensify in the coming years.

Medicare consists of four distinct parts: Part A (Hospital Insurance, or HI); Part B (Supplementary Medical Insurance, or SMI); Part C (Medicare Advantage, or MA); and Part D (the new prescription drug benefit added by the Medicare Prescription Drug, Improvement, and Modernization Act of 2003, or MMA). The program is administered by the Centers for Medicare and Medicaid Services (CMS).

This report provides an overview of Medicare. It begins with a capsule summary of key program features and major issues. This is followed by a more extensive discussion beginning with a brief program history, and then an outline of the key features of Parts A and B, also known as "Original Medicare." That is followed by overviews of Part C and Part D, a discussion of program financing, and a brief discussion of future program directions. Concluding sections include an overview of key program facts and a listing of CRS products that provide additional information on topics addressed in this report.

MEDICARE: A CAPSULE SUMMARY

Key Facts

- Nationwide health insurance program for aged (65 and over) and disabled
- 44.6 million people enrolled in FY2008
- Total outlays in FY2008: $459.4 billion
- Net outlays (not including beneficiary premiums) in FY2008: $389.9 billion

Program Structure

- "Original Medicare"
  - Parts A and B

- Medicare Advantage - alternative to "Original Medicare"
  - Part C

- Prescription Drug Benefits
  - Part D

"Original Medicare"

- 80% of beneficiaries get services through Parts A and B
- Part A and Part B - 2 different programs
  - Different eligibility requirements
  - Different benefits
  - Different beneficiary cost-sharing
  - Different financing

Eligibility

- Part A

- Almost all aged automatically eligible (they or their spouse paid payroll tax during working career)
- Disabled who have received cash disability payments for at least two years
- Persons with end stage renal disease (ESRD, kidney disease)

- Part B
  - Anyone who has Part A and all persons 65 and older
  - Voluntary - almost everyone enrolls

Benefits

- Part A
  - Inpatient hospital services
  - Post-hospital skilled nursing facility (SNF) services
  - Home health care (mostly post-hospital)
  - Hospice care

- Part B
  - Physicians services
  - Laboratory services
  - Therapy services
  - Specified preventive services
  - Outpatient hospital services
  - Durable medical equipment
  - Home health care (not covered under Part A)
  - Ambulance Services

Beneficiary Cost-Sharing

Part A

- Tied to "spell of illness" (starts with hospitalization and ends when out of hospital and SNF for 60 days)
- In each *spell of illness*, beneficiary pays:
  - Hospital care:
    - Deductible ($1,024 in 2008)
    - Days 61-90 - Daily charge ($256 in 2008)
    - Days 91-150 - Daily charge for lifetime reserve days ($512 in 2008)
    - Over 150 days - No coverage
  - Post Hospital SNF Care
    - Days 1 - 20: No cost-sharing
    - Days 21- 100: Daily coinsurance charge ($128 in 2008)

- Over 100 days - No coverage
- Home Health - No cost-sharing
- Hospice care - Nominal cost-sharing

Part B

- Annual Deductible - ($135 in 2008); and
- Coinsurance - 20% of Medicare's approved amount
- Exceptions:
  - Some services exempt from deductible and/or coinsurance
  - Mental health services: 50% cost-sharing
  - Hospital outpatient services: fixed amount which varies by service category

Payments for Services

- Payment rules under Part A and Part B differ for each service category and are quite complex
- Generally a pre-determined payment amount is established for a specific unit of service (such as a hospital stay)
- Typically, the law establishes annual update rules; however, they are frequently modified by Congress

Part C: Medicare Advantage (MA)

- 20% of beneficiaries get services through MA
- MA offers coordinated care and certain other private plan options for beneficiaries
- Voluntary for persons enrolled in both Part A and Part B
- MA enrollees get all their services through the plan
- Medicare makes a pre-determined monthly capitation payment to the MA plan for each beneficiary
- Capitation payments do not vary by amount of services used
- Federal government caps its liability (plans at risk for excess costs)

Part D: Drug Benefit

- New in 2006
- Voluntary
- Anyone who has Part A or Part B or enrolled in Part C can enroll
- Administered by private entities: MA plans and prescription drug plans (PDPs)
- Plans must meet minimum standards
- Plans compete to offer benefits in the region
- Beneficiaries select among plans

- Persons with incomes below 150% of poverty have assistance with premium and cost-sharing charges

Medicare Financing

Part A

- Financed primarily by payroll taxes paid by *current workers* and their employers:
  - Employees pay 1.45% on all earnings
  - Employers pay 1.45% on all earnings
  - Self-employed pay 2.9% on all earnings
- Revenues credited to Hospital Insurance (HI) trust fund

Part B

- Financed by a combination of beneficiary premiums and general revenues
  - 25% from monthly premiums ($96.40 in 2008) paid by current beneficiaries
  - 75% from general revenues
  - High income enrollees (in 2008, single beneficiaries with incomes over $82,000 and couples with incomes over $164,000) pay a higher premium
- Revenues credited to Supplementary Medical Insurance (SMI) trust fund

Part C

- No separate financing mechanism
- Payments to MA plans made in appropriate parts from HI and SMI trust funds
- Premiums, if any, vary by plan

Part D

- Financed by a combination of beneficiary premiums and general revenues
  - Beneficiaries pay different premiums depending on the plan they select
  - On average beneficiary premiums represent 25.5% of costs
  - General revenues finance the remainder
- Revenues credited to separate account in SMI trust fund

Financing: Key Points

- Part A financed almost entirely by current workers
- Part B and Part D financed by premiums paid by beneficiaries and general revenues (tax dollars)

- Pending insolvency discussion refers only to Part A (currently estimated to become insolvent in 2019)
- Parts B and D do not become insolvent because of the way they are financed

Current Concerns

- Medicare's overall growth rate not sustainable over time
  - Part A trust fund becomes insolvent
  - Parts B and D cost and premium increases will be substantial
- No easy solutions
- Some approaches focus on placing increasing reliance on private sector to deliver and manage benefits
- Other approaches focus on making changes within the current system

Medicare Trigger

- Enacted in 2003 as part of Medicare Modernization Act (MMA)
  - Intended to force consideration of reforms when there is "excess general revenue spending"
  - The law specifies that "excess spending" is reached when general revenues represent 45% or more of total program outlays
- Requirement for Medicare annual trustees report
  - Report required to specify if projected general revenue spending is expected to exceed 45% of outlays within seven years
  - President submits legislative proposal if finding is made for 2 successive years
  - Legislative proposal must contain recommendations to reduce percentage of total Medicare outlays funded by general revenues
  - Congress required to consider proposal on expedited basis.
  - Proposals to reduce the general revenue percentage can include increases in dedicated funding sources (primarily payroll taxes and premiums) and/or reductions in outlays for any part of the program.
- 2006 report contained finding
- 2007 report contained finding
- President submitted legislative proposal in February 2008
- Proposal would increase Part D premiums for higher income persons; incorporate value-based purchasing; and modify the medical liability system.
- In July 2008, the House approved a resolution specifying that the expedited parliamentary procedures required by MMA would not apply in the House for the remainder of the 110th Congress
- 2008 report also contained finding; submission of a legislative proposal will be required in February 2009
-

MEDICARE HISTORY

Medicare was enacted in 1965 (P.L. 89-97) in response to the concern that only about half of the nation's seniors had health insurance, and most of those only had coverage for inpatient hospital costs. The new program, which became effective July 1, 1966, included coverage for hospital and post-hospital services under Part A and doctors and other medical services under Part B. As was the case for the already existing Social Security program, Part A was to be financed by payroll taxes levied on current workers and their employers; persons had to pay into the system for 40 calendar quarters to become entitled to benefits. However, persons who turned 65 before 1968 were automatically covered, while those who turned 65 between 1967 and 1974 were covered under transitional provisions. Medicare Part B was voluntary; beneficiaries who elected to enroll would pay a monthly premium. Over 90% of the eligible population enrolled. Payments to health care providers under both Part A and Part B were to be based on the most common form of payment at the time, namely "reasonable costs" for hospital and other institutional services or "reasonable charges" for physicians and other medical services.

Medicare was considered a social insurance program, similar to Social Security. The 1965 law also established Medicaid, the federal/state health insurance program for the poor; this was an expansion of previous welfare-based assistance programs. Some low-income individuals qualified for both programs.

In the ensuing 40 years, the Medicare program has undergone considerable changes. P.L. 92-603, enacted in 1972, expanded program coverage to disabled individuals and to persons with end-stage renal disease (ESRD). This law also began to place limitations on the definitions of reasonable costs and reasonable charges. This was in order to gain some control over program spending which, even in the initial years, was in excess of the original projections.

During the 1980s and 1990s, a number of laws were enacted which included provisions designed to further stem the rapid increase in program spending and to postpone the bankruptcy of the Medicare Part A trust fund. This was typically achieved through tightening rules governing payments to providers of services and stemming the annual updates in such payments. The program moved from payments based on reasonable costs and reasonable charges to payment systems under which a pre-determined payment amount is established for a specified unit of service. At the same time, beneficiaries were given the option to obtain covered services through private managed care arrangements, typically health maintenance organizations. Most Medicare payment provisions were incorporated into larger budget reconciliation bills designed to control overall federal spending.

This effort culminated in the enactment of the Balanced Budget Act of 1997 (BBA 97, P.L. 105-33). This law slowed the rate of growth in payments to providers and established new payment systems for certain categories of providers. It also established the Medicare+Choice program, which expanded private plan options for beneficiaries and changed the way most plans were paid. BBA 97 further expanded preventive services covered by the program.

Subsequently, Congress became concerned that the BBA 97 cuts in payments to providers were somewhat larger than originally anticipated. Therefore, legislation was enacted in both 1999 (Balanced Budget Refinement Act of 1999, BBRA, P.L. 106-113) and

2000 (Medicare, Medicaid, and SCHIP Benefits Improvement and Protection Act of 2000, BIPA, P.L. 106-554) that was designed to mitigate the impact of BBA 97 on providers.

In 2003, Congress enacted a major Medicare bill, the Medicare PrescriptionDrug, Improvement, and Modernization Act of 2003 (MMA, P.L. 108-173). This legislation included the first major benefit expansion since 1965 and placed increasing emphasis on the private sector to deliver and manage benefits. It created a new voluntary outpatient prescription drug benefit to be administered by private entities. It also replaced the existing Medicare+Choice program with a new Medicare Advantage (MA) program; payments to these plans were increased in order to increase the availability of private plan options for beneficiaries. For the first time, MMA introduced the concept of income testing into Medicare. Low-income individuals get additional assistance under the new Part D drug program, while high income persons pay larger Part B premiums beginning in 2007. MMA also modified some provider payment rules and expanded covered preventive services. Finally, the legislation created a specific process for overall program review if general revenue spending exceeds a specified threshold.

During the 109th Congress, two laws were enacted that incorporated minor modifications to Medicare's payment rules. These were the Deficit Reduction Act of 2005 (DRA, P.L. 109-171) and the Tax Relief and Health Care Act of 2006 (TRHCA, P.L. 109-432). In the 110th Congress, additional changes were incorporated in the Medicare, Medicaid, and SCHIP Extension Act of 2007 (MMSEA, P.L. 110-173) and the Medicare Improvements for Patients and Providers Act of 2008 (MIPPA, P.L.110-275).

MEDICARE PARTS A AND B: "ORIGINAL MEDICARE"

Approximately 80% of Medicare beneficiaries receive covered services through Part A and Part B. The Part A and B structure, which remains to this day, reflects the political compromises made at the time of enactment in 1965. Together they are known as "Original Medicare." However, the two programs have different eligibility requirements, benefit structures, payment rules, and financing mechanisms. This section provides an overview of the key features of the two programs. (Medicare financing is discussed later in this report.)

Eligibility

Part A

Most persons age 65 or older are automatically entitled to Part A because they or their spouse paid Medicare payroll taxes for at least 10 years on earnings covered by either the Social Security or the Railroad Retirement systems.

Persons under age 65 who receive cash disability benefits from Social Security or the Railroad Retirement systems for at least 24 months are also entitled to Part A. (Since there is a five-month waiting period for cash payments, the Medicare waiting period is effectively 29 months.) The 24-month waiting period is waived for persons with amyotrophic lateral sclerosis (ALS, "Lou Gehrig's disease"). The disabled population also includes persons under age 65 with end stage renal disease (ESRD); coverage for these individuals generally begins in the fourth month of dialysis treatments or the month of a kidney transplant.

Persons over age 65 who are not automatically entitled to Part A may obtain coverage by paying a premium. The 2008 monthly premium is $423 ($233 for persons with at least 30 quarters of covered employment). In addition, disabled persons who lose their cash benefits solely because of higher earnings, and subsequently lose their extended Medicare coverage, may continue their Medicare enrollment by paying the premium.

Part B

Part B is voluntary. All persons entitled to Part A (and persons over 65 not entitled to Part A) may enroll in Part B by paying a monthly premium. The 2008 monthly premium is $96.40. Beginning in 2007, some higher-income individuals are paying higher premiums. (See the section on Financing, below.)

Persons who voluntarily enroll in Part A (because they are not automatically entitled to Part A) must also enroll in Part B. ESRD beneficiaries are also required to enroll in Part B.

Benefits and Beneficiary Cost-Sharing

Part A

Part A provides coverage for inpatient hospital services, post-hospital skilled nursing facility (SNF) services, post-hospital home health services, and hospice care, subject to certain conditions and limitations. Approximately 20% of Part A enrollees use Part A services during a year.

Inpatient Hospital Services

Coverage is linked to an individual's benefit period or "spell of illness"(defined as beginning on the day a patient enters a hospital and ending when he or she has not been in a hospital or SNF for 60 days). An individual admitted to a hospital more than 60 days after the last discharge from a hospital or SNF begins a new benefit period. Coverage in each benefit period is subject to the following conditions:

- Days 1-60. Beneficiary pays a deductible ($1,024 in 2008);
- Days 61-90. Beneficiary pays a *daily* coinsurance charge ($256 in 2008);
- Days 91-150. After 90 days, beneficiary may draw on one or more 60 lifetime reserve days, provided they have not been previously used.(Each of the 60 lifetime reserve days can be used only once during an individual's lifetime.) Beneficiary pays *daily* coinsurance charge ($512 in 2008).
- Days 151 and over. No coverage.

Inpatient mental health care in a psychiatric facility is limited to 190 days during a patient's lifetime.

Skilled Nursing Facility (SNF) Services

The program covers up to 100 days of post-hospital care for persons needing continued skilled nursing or rehabilitation services on a daily basis. The SNF stay must be preceded by a hospital stay of at least three days and the transfer to the SNF must occur within 30 days of the hospital discharge. There is no beneficiary cost-sharing for the first 20 days. Days 21-100 are subject tó *daily* coinsurance charges ($128 in 2008).

Home Health Services

Medicare covers visits by a home health agency when such services are required because an individual is confined to his or her home and needs skilled nursing care on an intermittent basis or physical therapy or speech language therapy. After establishing such eligibility, the continuing need for occupational therapy services may extend the eligibility period. Covered services include part-time or intermittent nursing care; physical or occupational therapy or speech language pathology services; medical social services; home health aide services; medical supplies and durable medical equipment. The services must be provided under a plan of care established by a physician and the plan must be reviewed by the physician at least every 60 days.

Home health services are covered under both Parts A and B. Part A covers up to 100 visits following a stay in a hospital or SNF. Part A also covers all home health services for persons not enrolled in Part B. All other home health services are covered under Part B. There is no beneficiary cost-sharing for home health services (though some other Part B services provided in connection with the visit, such as durable medical equipment, are subject to cost-sharing charges).

Hospice Care

Hospice services are provided to terminally ill Medicare beneficiaries with a life expectancy of six months or less for two 90-day periods followed by an unlimited number of 60-day periods. The individual's attending physician and the hospice physician must certify the need for the first benefit period, but only the hospice physician needs to recertify for subsequent periods. Hospice services are for the palliation and management of the illness and include drugs, and medical and support services. Hospice care is provided in lieu of most other Medicare services related to the curative treatment of the terminal illness. Beneficiaries electing hospice care from a hospice program may receive curative services for illnesses or injuries unrelated to their terminal illness and they may disenroll from the hospice at any time. Nominal cost-sharing is required for drugs and respite care.

Part B

Medicare Part B covers physicians' services, outpatient hospital services, durable medical equipment, and other medical services. Over 80% of Part B enrollees use Part B services during a year. The program generally pays 80% of the approved amount (generally a fee schedule or other predetermined amount) for covered services in excess of the annual deductible ($135 in 2008). The beneficiary is liable for the remaining 20%.

Most providers and practitioners are subject to limits on amounts they can bill beneficiaries for covered services. For example, physicians and some other practitioners may choose whether or not to accept "assignment" on a claim (namely to have the patient assign his or her right to payment to the physician). When a physician accepts assignment, the physician can only bill the beneficiary the 20% coinsurance plus any unmet deductible. When a physician agrees to accept assignment on all Medicare claims in a given year, the physician is referred to as a "participating physician." Physicians who do not agree to accept assignment on all Medicare claims in a given year are referred to as nonparticipating physicians. Nonparticipating physicians may or may not accept assignment for a given service. If they do not, they may charge beneficiaries more than the fee schedule amount on nonassigned claims; however, these "balance billing" charges are subject to certain limits.

For some providers, such as nurse practitioners and physician assistants, assignment is mandatory; these providers can only bill the beneficiary the 20% coinsurance and any unmet deductible. For other Part B services, such as durable medical equipment, assignment is optional; providers may bill beneficiaries for amounts above Medicare's recognized payment level and may do so without limit.

Covered Part B services include the following:

Physicians Services

Covered services include surgery, consultation, and home, office, and institutional visits. Certain limitations apply for services provided by chiropractors and podiatrists. Beneficiary cost-sharing for outpatient mental health treatment services equals 50% (rather than the usual 20%) of the approved amount.

Services of Non-Physician Practitioners

Covered services include those provided by physician assistants, nurse practitioners, certified registered nurse anesthetists, and clinical social workers.

Therapy Services

The program covers physical therapy and occupational therapy and speech language pathology services. The program establishes annual limits on covered services. The first is a $1,810 per beneficiary annual cap (in 2008) for all outpatient physical therapy services and speech language pathology services. The second is a $1,810 per beneficiary annual cap (in 2008) for all outpatient occupational therapy services. The limits, which are updated annually, apply to services provided by independent therapists as well as to those provided by comprehensive outpatient rehabilitation facilities (CORFs) and other rehabilitation agencies. The Secretary is required to implement an exceptions process, to be used in 2006, 2007, 2008, and 2009, for services meeting specified criteria for medically necessary services. The limits do not apply to outpatient services provided by hospitals.

Preventive Services

The program covers the following preventive services, at specified screening intervals. The regular Part B deductible and cost-sharing apply, except as otherwise specified.

- *"Welcome to Medicare" Physical Exam*. The program covers a onetime physical exam within the first six months of enrollment in Part B. Coverage is provided for a physical exam (not including clinical laboratory tests) and referral for preventive and other screening services covered under Part B. Effective January 1, 2009, the exam must be conducted during the first year rather than the first six months of enrollment and the deductible is waived.

- *Vaccines*. The program covers annual flu shots and pneumococcal vaccines (usually needed only once in a lifetime). No deductible or cost-sharing applies for these shots. The program also covers Hepatitis B vaccines for persons at medium to high risk for Hepatitis B.

- *Mammograms*. Annual screening mammograms are covered for asymptomatic women 40 and over. The deductible does not apply.

- *Pap Smears and Pelvic Exams*. Biennial exams are covered. More frequent tests may be covered under certain conditions. The deductible does not apply.

- *Colorectal cancer screening tests*. The following tests are covered for persons 50 and over (except no minimum age for screening colonoscopies):

    - Fecal Occult Blood Test — Once every 12 months;
    - Screening Flexible Sigmoidoscopy — Once every 48 months;
    - Screening Colonoscopy — Once every 10 years, but not within 48 months of a screening sigmoidoscopy; for high risk individuals once every 24 months;
    - Barium Enema — This test can substitute for a flexible sigmoidoscopy or colonoscopy; it is covered every 24 months for high risk individuals and every 48 months for other persons.
    - No cost-sharing applies for fecal occult blood test. The costsharing for flexible sigmoidoscopies and colonoscopies performed in hospital outpatient departments is 25%.

- *Prostate Cancer Screening*. The program covers annual screening tests for men aged 50 and over. Tests covered include a digital rectal exam and a prostate specific antigen (PSA) test. There is no deductible or cost-sharing for the PSA test.

- *Cardiovascular Screening*. Tests that check cholesterol and other blood fat (lipid) levels are covered once every five years.

- *Bone Mass Measurement.* The program covers the test once every 24 months for persons at risk for osteoporosis.

- *Diabetes Screening and Self-Management Training.* Screening tests may be covered up to twice a year for at-risk individuals; no deductible or cost-sharing applies. Diabetes self-management educational and training services are covered when furnished in an outpatient setting by a certified provider. The physician must certify the need for services and they must be provided under a comprehensive plan of care.

- *Glaucoma Tests.* They are covered annually for high-risk individuals.

- *Medical Nutrition Therapy (MNT) Services.* MNT services are covered for persons with diabetes or renal disease. The benefit includes an initial assessment of nutrition and lifestyle assessment; nutrition counseling; information regarding managing lifestyle factors that affect diet; and follow-up visits to monitor progress managing diet. Medicare covers 3 hours of one-on-one counseling services the first year, and 2 hours each year after that. If the beneficiary's condition, treatment, or diagnosis changes, he or she may be able to receive more hours of treatment with a physician's referral. A physician must prescribe these services and renew their referral yearly if continuing treatment is needed into another calendar year.

- *Ultrasound Screening for Abdominal Aortic Aneurysms.* Beginning January 1, 2007, coverage is provided under certain circumstances for persons with a family history or manifested risk factors. The deductible does not apply.

- *Additional Preventive Services.* Effective on or after January 1, 2009, these are services identified by the Secretary, subject to specified conditions.

Clinical Laboratory Tests; Diagnostic X-Ray Tests; Other Diagnostic Tests; and X-Ray, Radium, and Radioisotope Therapy

There is no coinsurance for clinical laboratory services.

Durable Medical Equipment (DME)

Coverage is provided for equipment that is durable, prescribed for use in the home, and primarily for medical purposes. It includes such items as: walkers, wheelchairs, hospital beds, and home oxygen equipment. Certain items require the doctor to complete a certificate of medical necessity. A power wheelchair or scooter is only covered if the doctor states that it is required, based on the patient's medical condition. DME must be obtained from a supplier enrolled in Medicare.

Prosthetic Devices

Coverage is provided for prosthetic devices (other than dental) which replace all or part of an internal body organ, braces, and artificial limbs and eyes. Also included are cataract glasses, contact lenses, or intraoccular lenses (IOLs) after cataract surgery with an intraoccular lens; patient pays any additional costs for insertion of presbyopia-correcting lens or for upgraded frame.

Drugs

Certain specified outpatient prescription drugs are covered under Medicare Part B. (However, most outpatient prescription drugs are covered under Part D, discussed below.) Covered Part B drugs include drugs furnished incident to physicians' services, immunosuppressive drugs following a Medicare-covered organ transplant, erythropoietin for treatment of anemia for persons with ESRD; oral anticancer drugs (provided they have the same active ingredients and are used for the same indications as chemotherapy drugs which would be covered if furnished incident to physicians services); and drugs needed for the effective use of DME.

Outpatient Hospital Services and Services in Ambulatory Surgical Centers (ASCs)

Coinsurance for outpatient hospital services can range as high as 40% of the payment amount; however, in no case can the amount exceed the inpatient hospital deductible ($1,024 in 2008). Regular cost-sharing applies for ASC services.

Home Health Services

Home health services not covered under Part A are covered under Part B. (See Part A discussion, above.)

Other Medical and Health Services

Additional covered services include ambulance services, home dialysis equipment and supplies, and services provided in rural health clinics (RHCs) and federally-qualified health centers (FQHCs).

Services for End-Stage Renal Disease Beneficiaries

Individuals with end stage renal disease (i.e., kidney disease) are eligible for all services covered under Parts A and B. In addition, they are covered for dialysis services and, when provided, kidney transplants.

Program Payments

When Medicare was first established, the program generally made payments on the basis of "reasonable costs" and "reasonable charges." However, program expenditures quickly began to exceed expectations. As a result, Congress sought to rein in expenditures by tightening payment rules. At first, limitations were placed on the definitions of reasonable costs and reasonable charges. Subsequently, the program moved toward payment systems under which a pre-determined payment amount is established for a specified unit of service, such as a hospital discharge or payment classification group. In 1983, the first prospective payment system (PPS) was established for inpatient hospital services, Medicare's largest spending category. Under the inpatient PPS (IPPS), the payment amounts are intended to represent the average cost for treating a patient for the same condition. Hospitals that are able to keep costs below the fixed payment are able to keep the difference, while those with costs exceeding the fixed payment lose money.

Over time, prospective payment and other pre-determined approaches, such as fee schedules, were established for a number of other service categories. The rules for each payment system are quite complex and differ for each system. Taken together, they are sometimes characterized as "*administered pricing*," since the price the government sets for the period does not fluctuate by supply or demand. The law generally specifies a formula for calculating an annual update to the payment amount, though Congress frequently amends the statutory requirements.

The following discussion is intended as only a brief overview of Medicare payment systems; for additional information, see CRS Report RL30526, *Medicare Payment Policies* and other CRS reports listed in the Appendix.

Inpatient Hospital Services

Short-Term General Hospitals

Medicare pays acute care hospitals using a prospectively determined payment for each discharge. A hospital's payment for its operating costs is the product of two components. The first component is a national standardized amount adjusted by a wage index associated with the area where the hospital is located or where it has been reclassified. The second component is the diagnosis related group (DRG) weight; this reflects the relative hospital resource use associated with the DRG to which the patient is assigned. DRGs are revised periodically, with the most recent update effective October 1, 2007. In that year, CMS began a two-year transition to a payment system that uses severity-adjusted DRGs. The new system has 335 base DRGs, most of which are split into two or three Medicare severity (MS) DRGs generally based on the presence of a comorbidity or complication. There are 743 MS-DRGs used for payment purposes.

Additional payments are made for: cases with extraordinary costs (outliers), indirect costs incurred by teaching hospitals for graduate medical education, and disproportionate share (DSH) costs for hospitals serving a disproportionate share of low-income patients. Additional payments may also be made for qualified new technologies that have been approved for special add-on payments. Note that physicians' services provided during an inpatient stay are paid under the physician fee schedule (discussed below), not under the IPPS system.

Payments are also made for capital costs. Medicare's capital IPPS is structured similarly to its operating IPPS for short-term general hospitals. A hospital's capital payment is based on a prospectively determined federal payment rate, depends on the DRG to which the patient is assigned, and is adjusted by a hospital's geographic adjustment factor. Qualified hospitals will receive indirect medical education and DSH adjustments to their capital payments as well. The teaching adjustment to capital payments is discontinued over the next two years.

Medicare makes payments outside the IPPS system for direct costs associated with graduate medical education costs for hospital residents, subject to certain limits. Medicare will also reimburse hospitals for 70% of the allowable costs associated with beneficiaries' unpaid deductible and copayment amounts.

Hospitals Receiving Special Consideration Under Medicare's IPPS

Special payment considerations may apply for hospitals meeting one of the following designations. Generally this results in higher payments than would apply under the IPPS system.

- *Sole Community Hospital (SCH)*. An SCH is a facility located in a geographically isolated area and deemed to be the sole provider of inpatient acute care hospital services in a geographic area based on distance, travel time, severe weather conditions, and/or market share as established by specific criteria.

- *Medicare Dependent Hospital (MDH)*. An MDH is a small rural hospital with a high proportion of patients who are Medicare beneficiaries. It cannot be an SCH and must have 100 or fewer beds.

- *Rural Referral Center (RRC)*. An RRC is a relatively large hospital, generally in a rural area, that provides a broad array of services and treats patients from a wide geographic area, as established by specific criteria.

IPPS Exempt Hospitals and Distinct Part Units

Certain hospitals or distinct hospital units are exempt from IPPS and paid on an alternative basis.

- *Inpatient Rehabilitation Facilities (IRFs)*. An IRF is a freestanding hospital or hospital-based distinct part unit that meets the modified "75% rule" and additional specified conditions. The rule specifies a minimum percentage of the IRF's inpatient population that must have at least one of the qualifying medical conditions. The compliance threshold to qualify for higher payments as an IRF (historically set at 75%) is set at 60% starting July 1, 2006. In order to be paid as an IRF, 60% of an entity's Medicare patients must have one of the qualifying medical conditions as either a primary or a secondary condition. Medicare payments to an IRF are made under a single PPS which covers both operating and capital costs. Payments will vary according to the case mix group (CMG) to which patients are assigned, based on their impairment level, functional status, comorbidity conditions, and age. Five CMGs are reserved for short-stay patients or those who die in the facility. Facility level adjustments such as the area wage index, rural location, share of low income patients, and teaching status would apply as well. Medicare's IRF-PPS also will provide additional payments for high cost outliers.

- *Long-Term Care Hospitals (LTCHs)*. An LTCH is an acute care general hospital that has a Medicare inpatient average length of stay greater than 25 days. An LTCH is paid on a discharge basis under an MS-DRG-based PPS which includes both operating and capital costs. The LTCH-PPS payment for a Medicare discharge is based on the patient's assignment into one of the covered MS-LTC-DRGs, as well as facility-specific adjustments.

- *Psychiatric Hospitals or Distinct Part Units*. Payments to an inpatient psychiatric facility (IPF) is based on a per diem PPS (IPFPPS). The system incorporates patient level adjustments for specified DRGs, as well as facility-level adjustments. Payments are higher in the earlier days of a stay.

- *Children's Hospitals and Cancer Hospitals*. These hospitals are paid on a reasonable cost basis, subject to certain limitations and, in certain cases, incentive payments.

- *Critical Access Hospitals (CAHs)*. A CAH is a limited-service facility that is: located more than 35 miles from another hospital (15 miles in certain circumstances); offers 24-hour emergency care; has no more than 25 acute care inpatient beds; and has a 96-hours or less average length of stay. As of January 1, 2006, states can no longer designate entities as necessary providers of care in order to qualify as a CAH. Certain grandfather provisions apply to those previously designated by the states. CAHs are paid on the basis of reasonable costs for inpatient, outpatient, and independent laboratory services; payments equal 101% of reasonable costs. A CAH may elect either a cost-based hospital outpatient service payment or an all-inclusive rate which is equal to a reasonable cost payment for facility services plus 115% of the fee schedule payment for professional (i.e. physicians') services.

Skilled Nursing Facility (SNF) Care

SNF services are paid under a PPS which is based on a per diem urban or rural base payment rate, adjusted for case mix and area wages. The per diem rate generally covers all services, including room and board, provided to the patient that day. The case-mix adjustment is made using the resource utilization groups (RUGs) system. The RUGs system uses patient assessments to assign a beneficiary to one of 53 categories and to determine the payment for the beneficiary's care. Patient assessments are done at various times during a patient's stay and the RUG category a beneficiary is placed in can change with changes in the beneficiary's condition. Extra payments are not made for extraordinarily costly cases ("outliers").

Home Health Services

Home health services are paid under a home health PPS, based on 60-day episodes of care; a patient may have an unlimited number of episodes. Under the PPS, a nationwide base payment amount is adjusted by differences in wages (using the hospital wage index). This amount is then adjusted for case mix using the applicable Home Health Resource Group (HHRG) to which the beneficiary has been assigned. The HHRG applicable to a beneficiary is determined following an assessment of the patient's condition and care needs using the Outcome and Assessment Information Set (OASIS); there are 80 HHRGs. Further payment adjustments may be made for outlier visits (for extremely costly patients), a significant change in a beneficiary's condition, a partial episode which occurs because a beneficiary transfers from one agency to another, or a low utilization adjustment for beneficiaries receiving four or fewer visits.

Hospice Care

Payment for hospice care is based on one of four prospectively determined rates (which correspond to four different levels of care) for each day a beneficiary is under the care of the hospice. The four rate categories are: routine home care, continuous home care, inpatient respite care, and general inpatient care. Payment rates are adjusted to reflect differences in area wage levels, using the hospital wage index. Payments to a hospice are subject to an aggregate cap that limits the average per beneficiary cost to a cap that is adjusted annually by changes to the medical care expenditure category of the CPI-U.

Physician Services and Other Services Paid Under the Physician Fee Schedule

A number of Part B services are paid under the physician fee schedule. These include services of physicians, nonphysician practitioners, and therapists. Most services described earlier as preventive services (except for laboratory tests paid under the laboratory fee schedule) and diagnostic tests are paid under the physician fee schedule. There are over 7,000 service codes under the fee schedule.

The fee schedule assigns relative values to each service code. These relative values reflect physician work (based on time, skill, and intensity involved), practice expenses, and malpractice expenses. The relative values are adjusted for geographic variations in the costs of practicing medicine. These geographically adjusted relative values are converted into a dollar payment amount by a national conversion factor. The conversion factor is updated each year by a formula specified in law. The update percentage equals the Medicare Economic Index (MEI, which measures inflation) subject to an adjustment to match spending under the cumulative sustainable growth rate (SGR) system which establishes a target for total expenditures since 1996. If total expenditures exceed the target, the update for a future year is reduced. Application of the SGR formula would have led to negative updates since 2002. However, Congress has acted several times to avert reductions, thereby overriding the statutory formula for the 2003-2009 period. The conversion factor for 2008 is 0.5% above that for 2007; the conversion factor for 2009 will be 1.1% above that for 2008. Unless Congress takes additional action, application of the SGR formula is expected to result in a sizeable reduction in the conversion factor in 2010 and continue to lead to annual reductions for the foreseeable future.

Additionally, physicians who report on selected quality measures for services for which quality measures are established will receive bonus payment for those services provided from July 2007-December 2010. The bonus payments are 1.5% during the second half of 2007 and 2008 and 2.0% for 2009 and 2010. Additional bonus payments will be made for 2009-2013 for Medicare professionals providing covered services who are successful electronic prescribers.

Clinical Diagnostic Laboratory Services

Clinical lab services are paid on the basis of area-wide fee schedules. There is a ceiling on payment amounts equal to 74% of the median of all fee schedules for the test. Fee schedule amounts are frozen through 2008. For the 2009-2013, the inflation update that would otherwise apply will be reduced by 0.5 percentage points each year

Durable Medical Equipment, Prosthetics and Orthotics (DMEPOS)

Except in competitive bidding areas described below, durable medical equipment (DME) is paid on the basis of a fee schedule. Items are classified into five groups for purposes of determining the fee schedules and making payments: (1) inexpensive or other routinely purchased equipment (defined as items costing less than $150 or which are purchased at least 75% of the time); (2) items requiring frequent and substantial servicing; (3) customized items; (4) oxygen and oxygen equipment; and (5) other items referred to as capped rental items. In general, fee schedule rates are established locally and are subject to national limits, with floors and ceilings. The floor is equal to 85% of the weighted average of all local payment amounts and the ceiling is equal to 100% of the weighted average of all local payment amounts.

Prosthetics and orthotics are also paid on the basis of a fee schedule in areas that are not competitive bidding areas. Fee schedule rates for prosthetics and orthotics, however, are established regionally and are subject to national limits which have floors and ceilings. The floor is equal to 90% of the weighted average of all regional payment amounts and the ceiling is equal to 120% of the weighted average of all regional payment amounts.

The fee schedules are generally updated annually by the CPI-U (Consumer Price Index), but Congress has often specified the reduction or elimination of updates in certain years.

MMA required the Secretary to establish a competitive bidding program for DMEPOS to replace the fee schedule payments. The program is required to be phased in, starting in 10 of the largest metropolitan statistical areas, expanding to 80 of the largest metropolitan areas, and remaining areas. The Secretary may first phase in items and services with the highest cost and highest volume, or those items and services that the Secretary determines to have the largest savings potential first. The Secretary may exclude certain areas from participation in the program. The program started on July 1, 2008; however, MIPPA terminated the first round of contracts, required the Secretary to rebid the first round in 2009, and delayed subsequent rounds of the program until 2011, in addition to other changes.

The DRA reduced the amount of time certain items of DME can be rented before ownership of the item is transferred to the beneficiary. For items in the capped rental category, such as hospital beds, nebulizers and wheelchairs, the rental period changed from a period not to exceed 15 months, to a maximum of 13 months; ownership of the equipment is then transferred to the beneficiary. For oxygen equipment, the rental period was limited in DRA to a maximum of 36 months. However, MIPPA eliminated the transfer-of-ownership requirement for oxygen equipment. After the 36-month rental period, the supplier retains ownership of the oxygen equipment but allows the beneficiary to continue using it. Medicare will continue to pay for oxygen refills and will pay for maintenance and servicing not covered by the manufacturer's warranty after the 36-month rental period.

Hospital Outpatient Department (HOPD) Services

Under the HOPD-PPS, the unit of payment is the individual service or procedure as assigned to an ambulatory payment classification (APC). To the extent possible, integral services and items (excluding physicians services paid under the physician fee schedule) are bundled within each APC. Specified new technologies are assigned to new technology APCs until clinical and cost data are available to permit assignment into a clinical APC. Medicare's payment for HOPD services is calculated by multiplying the relative weight associated with an APC by a conversion factor. For most APCs, 60% of the conversion factor is geographically adjusted by the IPPS wage index. Except for new technology APCs, each APC has a relative weight that is based on the median cost of services in that APC. The HOPD-PPS also includes pass-through payments for new technologies (specific drugs, biologicals, and devices) and payments for outliers. Starting in 2006, rural SCHs receive an additional 7.1% in Medicare payments. Special provisions apply for cancer hospitals, children's hospitals, small rural hospitals (that are not SCHs) with 100 or fewer beds, and SCHs with not more than 100 beds.

Ambulatory Surgical Center (ASC) Services

Beginning in January 2008, Medicare pays for surgery-related facility services provided in ASCs using a payment system based on the hospital OPPS (HOPD-PPS). The associated physician fees are paid using the physician fee schedule. Each of the 3,300 procedures approved for payment in an ASC is classified into an ambulatory payment classification (APC) group on the basis of clinical and cost similarity. Integral items and services are packaged with the primary service into an APC. Separate payments are made for corneal tissue acquisition, brachytherapy sources, certain radiology services, many drugs, and certain implantable devices. The ASC system uses the same payment groups (APCs) as the OPPS. The relative weights for most procedures in the ASC payment system is the same as the relative weights in the OPPS. The ASC system uses a conversion factor based on a percentage of the OPPS conversion factor. The percentage of this average dollar figure is set to ensure budget neutrality. By statute, total payments under the new ASC payment system should equal total payments under the old ASC payment system. A different payment method is used to set ASC payment for new, office based procedures, separately payable drugs, and deviceintensive procedures. New, office-based procedures are services that are performed in physician offices at least 50% of the time. Payment is set at the lower of the ASC rate or the practice expense portion of the physician fee schedule payment rate. This policy also applies to separably payable radiology services. Separately payable drugs in an ASC are paid the same amount as if provided in a hospital outpatient department. Different rules apply for device intensive procedures (where a device that is packaged into an APC accounts for more than half of its total payments). In general, CMS seeks to minimize the financial incentives to shift services from one setting (a physician office or hospital outpatient department) into an ASC.

Part B Covered Drugs and Vaccines

Medicare's payment for Part B covered drugs equals 106% of the average sales price.

Ambulance Services

Ambulance services are paid on the basis of a fee schedule. The fee schedule establishes seven categories of ground ambulance services and two categories of air ambulance services. The national fee schedule is fully phased in for air ambulance services. For ground ambulance services, payments through 2009 are equal to the greater of the national fee schedule or a blend of the national and regional fee schedule amounts. The portion of the blend based on national rates is 80% for 2007-2009. In 2010 and subsequently, the payments in all areas will be based on the national fee schedule amount.

' The payment for a service equals a base rate for the level of service plus payment for mileage. Geographic adjustments are made to a portion of the base rate. Additionally, the base rate is increased for air ambulance trips originating in rural areas and mileage payments are increased for all trips originating in rural areas. There is a 25% bonus on the mileage rate for trips of 51 miles and more.

Payments for ground ambulance services originating in rural areas are increased by 3%, and payments for such services originating in other areas are increased by 2% for the period July 1, 2008-December 31, 2009.

End-Stage Renal Disease (ESRD) Dialysis and Transplant Services

Dialysis services, paid for under Part B, are offered in three outpatient settings: hospital-based facilities, independent facilities, and the patient's home. There are two methods for payment. Under Method I, facilities are paid a prospectively set amount, known as the composite rate, for each dialysis session. Patients electing home dialysis may choose to be paid under either Method I or under Method II, as a series of separately billable services.

Under Method I, the composite rate is derived from audited cost data and adjusted for the national proportion of patients dialyzing at home versus in a facility, and for area wage differences. Beginning January 1, 2009, the payment rate for dialysis services will be "site neutral," and in applying the geographic index to providers of services, the labor share will be based on the labor share otherwise applied for renal dialysis facilities. Adjustments will no longer be made to the composite rate for hospital-based dialysis facilities to reflect higher overhead costs.

Beginning January 1, 2011, Medicare dialysis payments will be bundled (phased-in over four years) using a single payment for Medicare renal dialysis services that includes (1) items and services included in the composite rate as of December 31, 2010; (2) erythropoiesis stimulating agents (ESAs) for the treatment of ESRD; (3) other drugs and biologicals for which payment was made separately (before bundling); and (4) diagnostic laboratory tests and other items and services furnished to individuals for the treatment of ESRD.

Beneficiaries electing home dialysis may choose not to be associated with a acility and may make independent arrangements with a supplier for equipment, supplies, and support services. Payment to these suppliers, known as Method II, is made on the basis of reasonable charges, limited to 100% of the median hospital composite rate, except for patients on continuous cycling peritoneal dialysis, when the limit is 130% of the median hospital composite rate. The composite rate is case-mixed adjusted.

Kidney transplantation services, to the extent they are inpatient hospital services, are subject to the IPPS. However, kidney acquisition costs are paid on a reasonable cost basis.

MEDICARE PART C: MEDICARE ADVANTAGE (MA)

Approximately 20% of Medicare beneficiaries receive covered services through Part C, rather than through "Original Medicare." For a number of years, Medicare beneficiaries who are eligible for Medicare Part A and enrolled in Part B have had the option of obtaining covered services through private health plans. Under an agreement with CMS, a plan agrees to provide all services covered under Medicare Parts A and B (except for hospice care) in return for a capitated monthly payment. The same monthly payment is made regardless of how many or how few services a beneficiary actually uses. The plan is at-risk if costs, in the aggregate, exceed program payments; conversely, the plan can retain savings if costs are less than payments. In contrast, under the fee-for-service payment methodology used under "Original Medicare," a payment is made to a medical provider for each service (e.g., physician visit) or each unit of service (e.g., a hospital stay) provided.

Background

Medicare's first risk contract program was created in 1982. Under that program, private entities, mostly health maintenance organizations (HMOs), contracted with Medicare to provide covered services. The BBA, enacted in 1997, replaced the risk contract program with the Medicare+Choice (M+C) program. The M+C program established a new payment formula, which was designed both to reduce overall spending and to reduce the existing variation in payments to plans across the country. Following enactment of BBA 97, managed care plans began leaving the program, citing insufficient Medicare payments; however, other factors also played a role for some plans.

Subsequent legislation addressed some of the issues arising from passage of the BBA. Most recently, Congress made substantial changes to the M+C program with the passage of the MMA in 2003. The act created the Medicare Advantage (MA) program to replace the M+C program and introduced several provisions intended to increase the availability of private plans to Medicare beneficiaries. It provided for immediate payment increases to plans beginning in 2004. Beginning in 2006, it changed the payment structure for local plans and provided for the introduction of regional plans that operate like preferred provider organizations — a popular option in the private health insurance market. The legislation also provided financial incentives for plans to participate in this new regional option. Additionally, MA enrollees have access to the Part D drug benefit through their MA plan.

Beginning in 2010, the MA program will offer a six-year program (referred to as comparative cost adjustment) designed to test competition between local MA plans and fee-for-service Medicare, in limited areas.

Plan Types

There are several different types of plans that can qualify as MA plans. They include coordinated care plans (which includes health maintenance organizations and preferred provider organizations), private fee-for-service plans, Medical Savings Account plans, and certain other plan types operating under exceptions or demonstration authority. The following are the most common plan types available:

- *Health Maintenance Organizations (HMOs).* HMO plans offer services to plan members in designated service areas. Beneficiaries are generally required to obtain services from hospitals and doctors that are in the plan's network. Some plans offer a point-of-service option under which an individual may elect to obtain services from a non-network provider; in such cases, the individual pays more for the care. If the plan does not have a point of service option, the individual must pay out-of-pocket, except in emergency cases, for services provided by non-network providers.

- *Local Preferred Provider Organizations (PPOs).* Persons who enroll in PPOs are generally able to see any doctor or other provider that accepts Medicare. If enrollees use out-of-network (i.e. nonpreferred) providers, they will generally pay more, though the amount varies by plan. Local PPOs generally serve individual counties.

- *Regional PPOs (RPPOs).* Beginning in 2006, regional PPOs are available. Regional PPOs serve one or more of the 26 regions established by the Secretary. Each region consists of either a single state or multi-state area. MA regional plans cover both in- and out-of-network required services and have both a unified Part A and Part B deductible and a limit on out-of-pocket expenses; the limit varies by plan. This is the only group that has a specific limit on outof-pocket spending in connection with Part A and Part B services.

- *Special Needs Plans (SNPs).* A SNP may be any plan type (such as an HMO or PPO). However, unlike other plans, a SNP may, in accordance with regulations, restrict enrollment to special needs beneficiaries. Special needs beneficiaries are defined as MA eligible individuals who reside in long-term care facilities, who are eligible for both Medicare and Medicaid, or who meet requirements specified by the Secretary that identify people who would benefit from enrollment in a SNP for specified chronic or disabling conditions. SNPs may restrict enrollment for periods before January 1, 2011.Starting January 1, 2010, all new enrollees to a SNP must meet the definition of a special needs individual for the respective plan.

- *Private Fee-for-Service (PFFS) Plans.* A PFFS plan is one that (1) reimburses providers on a fee-for-service basis, (2) does not vary rates for a provider based on utilization, and (3) does not restrict the selection of providers who are lawfully authorized to provide services and agree to accept the terms and conditions of payment established by the plan. Starting in 2011, MIPPA require PFFS plans to establish contracted networks of providers in areas where two or more plans with networks (such as HMOs or local PPOs) serve Medicare beneficiaries starting in 2011. PFFS plans sponsored by an employer or union are required to establish contracted provider networks throughout their entire service area starting in 2011.

In general, MA organizations are required to offer at least one plan with Part D drug coverage. MA enrollees can only get Part D coverage through their MA plan. An exception applies for private fee-for-service plans; unlike most other MA plans, they are not required to offer Part D drug coverage, though they may elect to do so. Individuals in PFFS plans not offering drug coverage may purchase drug coverage through a stand-alone Part D drug plan.

Plan Enrollment

Beneficiaries newly eligible for Medicare Part A and enrolled in Part B can join an MA plan. Other persons can generally join an MA plan, or switch from one MA plan to another, only during the annual open enrollment period which occurs from November 15-December 31 each year. In addition, MA enrollees can generally change enrollment or drop out of their MA plans and return to Original Medicare during the first three months of each calendar year, or, for new enrollees, the first three months in which they are eligible to be enrolled in an MA plan. In certain cases, such as when an MA enrollee moves, he or she may switch plans at that time.

Payments to Plans

Payments to MA plans are based on a comparison of each plan's estimated cost of providing Medicare covered services (a bid) relative to the maximum amount the federal government is willing to pay for providing those services in the plan's service area (a benchmark). If a plan's bid is less than the benchmark, its payment will equal to its bid plus a rebate equal to 75% of the difference (between the benchmark and the bid). The rebate must be returned to the enrollees in the form of either additional benefits; reduced cost sharing; a reduction in the monthly Part B premium, prescription drug premium, or supplemental premium (for services beyond required Medicare benefits); or some combination of these options. The remaining 25% of the difference between the bid and the benchmark is retained by the federal government. If a plan's bid is equal to or above the benchmark, its payment will be the benchmark amount and each enrollee in that plan will pay an additional premium, equal to the amount by which the bid exceeds the benchmark.

Each year, plans wishing to participate in the MA program must submit new bids. The Secretary has the authority to negotiate the bid amounts, except for PFFS plans. Benchmark amounts are increased each year by the greater of either 2% or growth in overall Medicare. In years specified by the Secretary, a benchmark for an area can be set at per capita spending in original Medicare if that amount is greater than the benchmark the area would otherwise receive.

Beginning in 2006, the MA program began to offer MA regional plans. Like local plans, regional plans must submit bids to the Secretary that, in relation to the benchmark, determine the payment the plan receives for each enrollee. The regional program is different from the local program in that the plan bids help determine the benchmarks for each region. The regional benchmarks include two components: (1) a statutorily determined amount (comparable to benchmarks described above), and (2) a weighted average of plan bids. Thus, a portion of the benchmark is competitively determined. Similar to local plans, plans with bids below the benchmark will be given a rebate while plans with bids above the benchmark will require an additional enrollee premium.

Additional financial incentives are provided to encourage regional plan participation. During 2006 and 2007, Medicare shared risk with an MA regional plan if its costs fell above or below a statutorily-specified risk corridor. Starting in 2014, a stabilization fund is available to provide incentives for regional plans to enter into or to remain in the MA program. Due to changes in MIPPA, the stabilization fund is financed entirely with a portion of the savings from the regional plan bidding process.

PART D: OUTPATIENT PRESCRIPTION DRUGS

As noted, MMA added a new voluntary outpatient prescription drug benefit, beginning in 2006. Coverage is provided through private prescription drug plans (PDPs) or MA prescription drug (MA-PD) plans. The program relies on these private plans to provide coverage and to bear some of the financial risk for drug costs; federal subsidies covering the bulk of the risk is provided to encourage participation.

Unlike other Medicare services, the benefits can only be obtained through private plans. Further, while all plans have to meet certain minimum requirements, there are significant differences among them in terms of benefit design, drugs included on plan formularies (i.e. list of covered drugs) and cost-sharing applicable for particular drugs.

Eligibility and Plan Enrollment

Each individual enrolled in Part A or Part B is entitled to obtain qualified prescription drug coverage through enrollment in a prescription drug plan. A beneficiary enrolled in an MA plan providing qualified prescription drug coverage (MA-PD plan) obtains coverage through that plan. In general, MA enrollees can not enroll in a stand-alone prescription drug plan under Part D.

Medicare beneficiaries enrolled in Part A or Part B on or before January 31, 2006, had to enroll by May 15, 2006; those eligible in February 2006 had until May 31, 2006. Those eligible for Medicare beginning March 2006 or later have an initial seven-month enrollment period beginning three months before the month of Medicare eligibility. This initial eligibility period is the same as that applicable for Medicare Part B.

An individual who does not enroll during his or her initial enrollment period is only able to enroll during the annual open enrollment period, which occurs from November 15-December 31 each year. Coverage begins the following January 1. Persons who fail to enroll during their initial enrollment period are subject to a penalty if they decide to enroll in the program at a later date. However, they are not subject to the penalty if they have maintained "creditable" drug coverage through another source. One source of possible creditable coverage is retiree health coverage offered by a former employer or union.

Special rules apply for persons who qualify for the low-income subsidy. These persons are not subject to the delayed enrollment penalty otherwise applicable to persons who miss the enrollment deadline.

Benefits

Qualified Part D plans are required to offer either "standard coverage" or alternative coverage, with actuarially equivalent benefits. In 2008, "standard coverage" has a $275 deductible, 25% coinsurance for costs between $276 and $2,510. From this point, there is no coverage until the beneficiary has out-of-pocket costs of $4,050 ($5,726.25 in total spending); this coverage gap has been labeled the "doughnut hole." Once the beneficiary reaches the catastrophic limit, the program pays all costs except for nominal cost-sharing.

Most plans offer actuarially equivalent benefits rather than the standard package. A number of plans have reduced or eliminated the deductible. Many plans offer tiered cost-sharing under which lower cost-sharing applies for generic drugs, higher costsharing applies for preferred brand name drugs, and even higher cost-sharing applies for non-preferred brand name drugs. Some plans provide some coverage in the doughnut hole; this is generally limited to generic drugs.

Low-Income Provisions

A major focus of the drug benefit is the enhanced coverage provided to low-income individuals who enroll in Part D. Low-income enrollees, including persons (known as "dual eligibles"- those persons enrolled in both Medicare and Medicaid) who previously received drug benefits under Medicaid, have their prescription drug costs paid under the new Part D. Persons with incomes below 150% of poverty have assistance with some portion of their premium and costsharing charges. Persons with the lowest incomes have the highest level of benefits.

Drug Payments

Plans determine payments for drugs and are expected to negotiate prices. The federal government is prohibited from interfering in the price negotiations between drug manufacturers, pharmacies, and plans (the so-called "non-interference clause").

Interaction with Retiree Plans

MMA included significant incentives for employers to continue to offer coverage to their retirees. Specifically, special federal subsidy payments are made to employers or unions offering drug coverage at least actuarially equivalent to "standard coverage." Subsidy payments are made on behalf of an individual covered under a retiree plan who is eligible to enroll under a PDP or MA-PD plan, but elects not to. In 2008, subsidy payments equal 28% of the retiree's gross drug costs between $275 and $5,600. The federal government is not taking the subsidy in behalf of persons enrolled in TRICARE or the federal employees health benefits (FEHB) program.

Employers or unions may select an alternative option (instead of taking the subsidy) with respect to Part D. They may elect to pay a portion of the Part D premiums. They may also elect to provide enhanced coverage, though this has some financial consequences for the employer or union. Enhanced coverage may be provided through supplementary or "wrap around" benefits. Alternatively, employers or unions may contract with a PDP or MA-PD to offer the coverage. Finally, they may become a Part D plan sponsor themselves for their retirees.

MEDICARE ADMINISTRATION

At the federal level, Medicare is administered by the Centers for Medicare and Medicaid Services (CMS) within the Department of Health and Human Services (HHS). Day-to-day program operations, including processing benefits and paying claims, are conducted by private Medicare contractors. Fiscal intermediaries (FIs) perform claims administration functions for Part A services and Part B services performed by Part A providers (such as hospitals and skilled nursing facilities). Carriers perform claims administration functions for other Part B services. Day-to-day program operations for MA plans, MA-PD plans, and PDPs are handled by the plans themselves.

Under contracting reform, mandated by the MMA, the Secretary is authorized to replace FIs and carriers with 19 competitively-selected, Medicare Administrative Contractors (MACs) by 2011. Fifteen A/B MACs will perform claims processing operations for Part A and B Medicare providers. The four regional carriers (DMERCs), which previously handled all durable medical equipment claims in the country, were transitioned to DME MACs. As of December 2007, 1 A/B MAC and the 4 DME MACs were fully operational.

CMS also contracts with private organizations to conduct other administrative functions such as detecting and collecting improper payments, investigating alleged fraud and abuse, and ensuring the quality of care provided to Medicare beneficiaries.

MEDICARE FINANCING

Medicare is financed from three principal sources, namely payroll taxes, general revenues, and premiums paid by beneficiaries. Different revenue sources are directed to specific Parts of the program.

Medicare's financial operations are accounted for through two trust funds, the Hospital Insurance (HI) trust fund and the Supplementary Medical Insurance (SMI) trust fund, which are maintained by the Department of the Treasury. The HI and SMI trust funds are overseen by a board of trustees that makes annual reports to Congress.

The trust funds are an accounting mechanism; there is no actual transfer of money into and out of a fund. Income to the trust funds is credited to the fund in the form of interest-bearing government securities. Expenditures for services and administrative costs are recorded against the fund. The securities represent obligations that the government has issued to itself. As long as the trust fund has a balance, the Treasury Department is authorized to make payments for it from the U.S. Treasury.

Part A Financing

The primary source of funding for Part A is payroll taxes paid by employees and employers. Each pays a tax of 1.45% on earnings; the self-employed pay 2.9%. Unlike Social Security, there is no upper limit on earnings subject to the tax. Other sources of income include (1) a portion of federal income taxes that individuals pay on their social security benefits; (2) premiums paid by voluntary enrollees who are not automatically entitled to Medicare Part A through their (or their spouse's) work in covered employment; (3) government credits; and 4) interest on federal securities held by the trust fund. Income for Part A is credited to the HI trust fund.

Part B Financing

Medicare Part B is financed through a combination of beneficiary premiums and federal general revenues. Beneficiary premiums equal 25% of estimated program costs for the aged. (The disabled pay the same premium as the aged.) Federal general revenues account for the remaining 75%. Income for Part B is credited to the SMI trust fund.

The 2008 monthly Part B premium is $96.40. Individuals receiving Social Security benefits have their Part B premium payments automatically deducted from their Social Security benefit checks. An individual's Social Security check cannot go down from one year to the next as a result of the annual Part B premium increase (except in the case of higher income individuals subject to income-related premiums).

Since the inception of Medicare, all Part B enrollees paid the same Part B premium, regardless of their income level. For many years, Congress debated whether or not it was appropriate for taxpayers to pay (through general revenue financing) three-quarters of Part B costs for higher income persons, since low income and middle income working persons might be subsidizing higher income elderly persons.

In response, Congress included a provision in MMA that required higher income enrollees to pay higher premiums beginning in 2007. In 2008, individuals whose modified adjusted gross income (AGI) in 2006 exceeded $82,000 and couples whose modified AGI exceeded $164,000 are subject to higher premium amounts. In 2008, they pay total premiums ranging from 31.7% to 61.7% of the value of Part B. When fully phased-in in 2009, higher income individuals will pay total premiums ranging from 35% to 80% of the value of Part B.

CMS estimates that 5% of enrollees will pay the higher premiums in 2008. For singles, the higher monthly premium amounts are $122.20 for beneficiaries with incomes (in 2006) over $82,000 and less than or equal to $102,000, $160.90 for incomes over $102,000 and less than or equal to $153,000, $199.70 for incomes greater than $153,000 and less than or equal to $205,000, and $238.40 for incomes greater than $205,000. For couples filing joint tax returns, the premium amounts are $122.20 for beneficiaries with incomes over $164,000 and less than or equal to $204,000, $160.90 for incomes over $204,000 and less than or equal to $306,000, $199.70 for incomes greater than $306,000 and less than or equal to $410,000, and $238.40 for incomes greater than $410,000.

Part C Financing

Payments for spending under the Medicare Advantage program are made in appropriate parts from the HI and SMI trust funds. There is no separate trust fund for Part C.

Part D Financing

Medicare Part D is financed through a combination of beneficiary premiums and federal general revenues. In addition, certain transfers are made from the states. These transfers, referred to as "clawback payments," represent a portion of the amounts states could otherwise have been expected to pay for drugs under Medicaid if drug coverage for the dual eligible population had not been transferred to Part D. Part D revenues are credited to a separate Part D account within the SMI trust fund.

Beneficiaries pay different premiums depending on the plan they have selected (and whether or not they are entitled to low-income premium subsidies). On average, beneficiary premiums account for 25.5% of expected total Part D costs for basic coverage. Part D premium payments may be automatically deducted from Social Security benefit checks, paid directly to the PDP sponsor or MA-PD organization, or made through an electronic funds transfer.

Medicare Solvency

When people refer to the pending insolvency of Medicare, they are actually referring to the pending insolvency of the HI trust fund. Medicare trustees define insolvency as occurring when trust fund assets at the beginning of the year are insufficient to pay program benefits for the forthcoming year. Because of the way it is financed, the SMI fund (including the Part D account) does not face insolvency although its rapid growth rate is a drain on federal spending. Further, continued premium increases may place a financial burden on some beneficiaries.

The 2008 trustees report projects that under intermediate assumptions, the HI trust fund will become insolvent in 2019. The report further states that beginning in 2004, tax income (from payroll taxes and from the taxation of Social Security benefits) began to fall below expenditures. Expenditures exceed *total* income each year beginning in 2008 (except for 2009). If income falls short of expenditures, costs are met by drawing on HI fund assets through transfers from the general fund of the Treasury until the fund is depleted.

45% Trigger

The rapid increases in total Medicare costs has long been of concern to Congress and others. The trustees have emphasized the importance of examining the program as a whole, rather than just the HI trust fund. Of particular concern is the fact that over time the economy will be unable to support the increasing reliance on general revenues, which in large measure come from taxes paid by the under-65 population. In response, MMA required the annual trustees report to include an expanded analysis of Medicare expenditures and revenues. Specifically, each year the trustees must determine whether general revenue financing will exceed 45% of total Medicare outlays within the next seven years. General revenue financing is defined as: total Medicare outlays minus dedicated financing sources (i.e., HI payroll taxes; income from taxation of Social Security benefits; state transfers for prescription drug benefits; premiums paid under Parts A, B, and D; and any gifts received by the trust funds).

If the trustees determine that general revenue financing will exceed 45% of total financing within seven years, an finding of "excess general revenue funding" is made." The 2006 report projected 'that the 45% level would first be exceeded in FY2012; the 2007 report projected that it would first be exceeded in 2013. Both findings were within the required seven-year test period. Both reports therefore, made a determination of "excess general revenue funding."

MMA requires that if an excess general revenue funding determination is made for two successive years, the President is required to submit a legislative proposal to respond to the warning. The proposal must be submitted, within 15 days of submission of the next President's Budget (unless during the intervening period legislation is enacted, which eliminates such excess general revenue funding). Since warnings were issued in 2006 and 2007, the proposal was due within 15 days of submission of the President's FY2009 budget in early 2008.

The President submitted the required proposal in February 2008. It included provisions to increase Part D premiums for higher income persons; incorporate value-based purchasing; and modify the medical liability system. The Congress was required to consider the proposal on an expedited basis, though passage of legislation within a specific time frame was not required. On July 24, 2008, the House of Representatives adopted a resolution which provides that the expedited parliamentary procedures contained in MMA shall not apply in the House during the remainder of the 110th Congress.

The 2008 trustees report also contained a funding warning. Therefore the President will be required to submit a legislative proposal early in 2009.

ADDITIONAL INSURANCE COVERAGE

Medicare provides broad protection against the costs of many, primarily acute care, services. However, the program does not cover all services which may be used by its aged and disabled beneficiaries. Medicare does not cover eyeglasses, hearing aids, dentures, or most long-term care services. Further, unlike most private insurance polices, it does not include an annual "catastrophic" cap on out-of-pocket spending on cost-sharing charges for services covered under Parts A and B (except for persons enrolled in regional PPOs under MMA). Prior to implementation of the drug benefit in 2006, the program generally covered only about one-half of beneficiaries' total health care expenses. (More recent data are not available.)

Most Medicare beneficiaries have some coverage in addition to Medicare. The following are the main sources of additional coverage for Medicare enrollees.

- *Medicare Advantage.* Many MA plans offer services in addition to those covered under Original Medicare.

- *Employer Coverage.* Coverage may be provided through a current or former employer. In recent years, a number of employers have cut back on the scope of retiree coverage. Some have dropped such coverage entirely, particularly for future retirees. As noted earlier, the MMA attempted to stem this trend by offering subsidies to employers who offer drug coverage, at least as good as that available under Part D. (See discussion, above.)

- *Medigap.* Individual insurance policies which supplement Medicare are referred to as Medigap policies. Beneficiaries with Medigap insurance typically have coverage for a portion of Medicare's deductibles and coinsurance; they may also have coverage for some items and services not covered by Medicare. Individuals generally select one of the standardized plans, though not all plans are offered in all states.

- *Medicaid.* Certain low-income Medicare beneficiaries may also be eligible for full or partial benefits under their state's Medicaid program. Persons eligible for the full range of benefits (known as the "full dual eligibles") generally have the majority of their health care expenses met through a combination of coverage under the two programs; Medicare pays first, with Medicaid picking up most of the remaining costs. Certain other individuals are entitled to more limited protection under one of three Medicaid Savings programs. The Qualified Medicare Beneficiary (QMB) program pays Medicare Part B premiums and Medicare cost-sharing charges for persons under 100% of poverty. The Specified Low-Income Medicare Beneficiary (SLMB) program pays Part B premium charges for those between 100% and 120% of poverty, while the Qualified Individual (QI) program pays such premiums for those between 120% and 135% of poverty.

- *Other Public Sources.* Individuals may have additional coverage through the Department of Veterans Affairs, or TRICARE for military retirees eligible for Medicare (and enrolled in Part B).

In the years prior to implementation of the drug benefit, close to 90% of beneficiaries had some form of additional coverage. (Some persons may have had more than one type of such coverage.) More recent information is not available.

MEDICARE DIRECTIONS

The Medicare program is likely to be the subject of continuing review for a number of years. Both Congress and the Medicare trustees continue to register concern about the rapid rise in Medicare spending and the ability of existing funding mechanisms to support the program over the long-term. Only the Part A fund faces an actual insolvency date. However, few observers believe that the program's total growth rate is sustainable over time. The 2008 trustees report noted that total program expenditures, which represented 3.1% of GDP in 2006, were expected to climb to 7.0% by 2035 and rise to 10.7% by 2080. It further noted that the level of program expenditures is expected to exceed that for Social Security in 2028 and be 85% more than the cost of that program by 2082.

A combination of factors have contributed to the rapid increase in Medicare costs. These include increases in overall medical costs, advances in health care delivery and medical technology, increases in the percentage of the population over 65, and longer life spans. The trend is expected to accelerate in 2011 when the baby boom generation (persons born between 1946 and 1964) begin to turn 65 and become eligible for Medicare. The issues confronting the program are not new, nor are the possible responses likely to get any easier. Solutions involve raising taxes, cutting benefits, raising beneficiaries' out-of-pocket costs, or some combination of these approaches. Members of Congress, Medicare trustees, and many other observers continue to warn that the problems need to be addressed. At the same time, some Members and beneficiary advocates express concern about the potential impact of any solution on beneficiaries' out-of-pocket costs or access to needed services.

It seems likely that in the short-term, Congress will focus its attention on specific Medicare issues, for example physician payment updates. It may also consider Medicare spending reductions as part of legislation (such as budget reconciliation) designed to reduce overall federal spending below specified levels over a specific time period.

At the same time, the Administration, Congress and others may also examine a broad range of policy options designed to achieve more long term reforms. For a number of years, various options have been suggested; however, there is no consensus on the approach that should be taken. One option is placing increasing reliance on the private sector to deliver and manage benefits. This is the approach first used for managed care options under Part C. More recently, the new Part D drug benefit gave increased flexibility to private entities. Within federally-established parameters, individual entities design their benefit packages and determine payment amounts. The intention is to encourage competition by allowing beneficiaries to select coverage that best meets their needs. Proponents claim that this will result in lower overall costs as well as enable the federal government to distance itself from the business of establishing detailed payment rules for each service category.

Some Members and other observers oppose the efforts to change the basic structure of Medicare. They contend that a single nationwide benefit structure, administered by the federal government, has served beneficiaries well and should be retained. They contend that any necessary savings for Part A and B services can be achieved within the context of the existing program and suggest that increased MA payments have actually increased overall program costs. Additionally, some persons also suggest that savings could be achieved under Part D if the federal government were allowed to enter into price negotiations with drug manufacturers.

At one time, it was thought that the MMA provision relating to an excess general revenue funding determination might have an impact on the Medicare discussion this year. For the second straight year, the Medicare trustees report had contained an excess general revenue funding determination under which general revenues are expected to be greater than 45% of outlays within the next seven years. (See "Financing" section, above.) As a result, the President was required to submit a legislative proposal responding to the warning. The President submitted the proposal in February 2008. MMA had required expedited congressional action. However, on July 24, 2008, the House of Representatives adopted a resolution which provides that the expedited parliamentary procedures contained in MMA shall not apply in the House during the remainder of the 110th Congress.

The 2008 trustees report also contained a funding warning. Therefore, under the MMA provisions, the President will be required to submit a legislative proposal early in 2009.

It should be noted that the MMA provision defines general revenues as total outlays minus dedicated revenues (primarily payroll taxes and premiums). Under this calculation, increases in dedicated revenues and/or reductions in outlays in any part of Medicare will lower general revenues and can be used to meet the trigger requirements. It should be noted that lowering Part A spending lowers both overall Medicare spending and "excess general revenue spending." However, if no other changes were made, spending under Parts B and D (and associated general revenue financing) would represent a larger proportion of total spending.

On the other hand, legislation directed at general revenue financing under Parts B and D will not address the pending insolvency of Part A which is funded primarily by payroll taxes. It is therefore expected that Congress will need to examine a variety of options in the coming years.

KEY MEDICARE STATISTICS

Tables 1-3 show CBO estimates from the March 2008 Medicare Fact Sheet which contains information on the various components of program spending. CBO March baseline numbers are the numbers Congress uses when it considers legislation. Slightly different estimates are provided by the Medicare trustees.

Table 1. Medicare Outlays, Selected Years ($ in billions)

	FY2008	FY2009	FY2013	FY2018
Total Outlays	$459.4	$491.5	$642.0	$894.6
Offsetting Receipts (premiums and amounts paid by states)	69.4	72.2	90.3	128.0
Net Outlays	389.9	419.3	551.7	766.6

Source: Congressional Budget Office (CBO), Fact Sheet for CBO's March 2008 Baseline: Medicare.
Note: Totals may not add due to rounding.

Table 2. Distribution of Total Outlays ($ in billions)

	FY2008		FY2009	
	Amount	Percent	Amount	Percent
Benefits	$452.5	98.5	$484.7	98.6
Part A	225.3	49.0	240.3	48.9
Part B	181.9	39.6	190.2	38.7
Part D	45.5	9.9	54.3	11.0
Administration	7.0	1.5	6.9	1.4
Total	459.4	100.0	491.5	100.0

Source: Congressional Budget Office (CBO), Fact Sheet for CBO's March 2008 Baseline: Medicare.
Notes: Spending for Part C is made in appropriate parts from the Part A and B trust funds and is recorded under benefits totals for Part A or B. Totals may not add due to rounding.

Table 3. Medicare Benefit Payments, by Category ($ in billions)

	FY2008	FY2009
Total	**$452.5**	**$484.7**
Part A, only	166.2	171.3
Hospital Inpatient Care	132.2	135.9
Skilled Nursing Facilities	22.9	23.5
Hospice	11.1	11.9
Part B, only	122.1	120.7
Physician Fee Schedule	56.4	52.6
Other Professional and Outpatient Ancillary	28.9	30.0
Other Facility Services	16.6	16.6
Hospital Outpatient	20.2	21.5
Parts A and B	110.5	130.1
Group Plans	94.1	112.8
Home Health Agencies	16.4	17.3
	FY2008	**FY2009**
Part D	45.4	54.3
Payment to Prescription Drug Plans	25.1	32.2
Payments to Union/Employer-sponsored	3.2	3.3
Low-Income Subsidy Payments	17.1	18.8
Recoveries[a]	8.3	8.2

Source: Congressional Budget Office (CBO), Fact Sheet for CBO's March 2008 Baseline: Medicare.
Note: Totals may not add due to rounding.
a. Amounts paid to providers and later recovered

Table 4. Projected Growth in Medicare Population (in millions)

	FY2008 (est)	FY2013 (est.)	FY2018 (est.)
Total (Part A enrollment)	44.0	49.4	57.2

Source: Congressional Budget Office (CBO), Fact Sheet for CBO's March 2008 Baseline: Medicare.

Table 5. Characteristics of Medicare Population, 2002 (by percent)

Race	100	**Age**	100
White (not Hispanic or Latino)	78.2	Aged	84.8
Black (not Hispanic or Latino)	9.6	65-74	43.8
Hispanic or Latino	7.5	75-84	29.8
Other	4.7	85 and over	11.2 .
Sex	100	**Disabled**	15.2
Male	44.1	Under 45	3.8
Female	55.9	45-64	11.4

Source: Department of Health and Human Services, Centers for Disease Control and Prevention, National Center for Health Statistics, Health, United States 2007, November 2007, p. 411. [http://www.cdc.gov/nchs/data/hus/hus07.pdf]
Note: Totals may not add due to rounding.

**Table 6. Percentage of Persons Age 65 and Over Characterized as
Poor or Near Poor, 2005**

	Poor[a]	Near Poor[a]
All Races and Origins	10.1	26.7
Hispanic or Latino	19.9	34.7
Black or African American, only	23.3	34.5
Asian only	12.8	20.1
White only, not Hispanic or Latino	7.9	25.4

Source: Department of Health and Human Services, Centers for Disease Control and Prevention, National Center for Health Statistics, Health, United States 2007, November 2007, p. 97. [http://www.cdc.gov/nchs/data/hus/hus07.pdf].

Note: Includes some aged persons not enrolled in Medicare; does not include the disabled.

a. Poor is defined as family income less than 100% of the poverty level and near poor is defined as family income between 100% and 199% of the poverty level. Assets are not considered.

APPENDIX: OTHER CRS PRODUCTS

Recent Legislation

- CRS Report RL34592, *P.L.110-275: The Medicare Improvements for Patients and Providers Act of 2008,* by Hinda Chaikind, Jennifer O'Sullivan, Sibyl Tilson, Paulette Morgan, Holly Stockdale, Jim Hahn, Gretchen A. Jacobson, Richard Rimkunas, Evelyne Baumrucker, April Grady, Jean Hearne, Elicia J. Herz, Julie Stone, Gene Falk, and Emile Stoltfus

- CRS Report RL34360, *P.L. 110-173: Provisions in the Medicare, Medicaid, and SCHIP Extension Act of 2007,* by Hinda Chaikind, Jim Hahn, Jean Hearne, Elicia J. Herz, Gretchen A. Jacobson, Paulette C. Morgan, Chris L. Peterson, Holly Stockdale, Jennifer O'Sullivan, Julie Stone, and Sibyl Tilson

- CRS Report RL33131, *Budget Reconciliation FY2006: Medicaid, Medicare, and State Children's Health Insurance Program (SCHIP)* Provisions, by Evelyne P. Baumrucker, Hinda Chaikind, April Grady, Jim Hahn, Jean Hearne, Elicia J. Herz, Bob Lyke, Paulette C. Morgan, Jennifer O'Sullivan, Richard Rimkunas, Julie Stone, Sibyl Tilson, and Karen Tritz

- CRS Report RL31966, *Overview of the Medicare Prescription Drug, Improvement, and Modernization Act of 2003 (MMA),* by Jennifer O'Sullivan, Hinda Chaikind, Sibyl Tilson, JenniferBoulanger, and Paulette C. Morgan

- CRS Report RL32005, *Medicare Fee-for-Service Modifications and Medicaid Provisions of H.R. 1 as Enacted,* (MMA provisions) by Sibyl Tilson, Jennifer Boulanger, Jean Hearne, Steve Redhead, Evelyne Baumrucker, Julie Stone, Bernadette Fernandez, and Karen Tritz

In General

- CRS Report RL30526, *Medicare Payment Policies*, by Sibyl Tilson, Hinda Chaikind, Jennifer O'Sullivan, Julie Stone and Paulette C. Morgan
- CRS Report RL34359, *Medicare: FY2009 Budget Issues*, by Hinda Chaikind, Jim Hahn, Gretchen A. Jacobson, Paulette C. Morgan, Jennifer O'Sullivan, Holly Stockdale, Julie Stone, and Sibyl Tilson
- CRS Report RL33713, *Pay-for-Performance in Health Care*, by Jim Hahn
- CRS Report RL33587, *Medicare Secondary Payer — Coordination of Benefits*, by Hinda Chaikind
- CRS Report RL31223, *Medicare: Supplementary "Medigap" Coverage*, by Jennifer O'Sullivan
- CRS Report RL34217, *Medicare Program Integrity: Activities to Protect Medicare from Payment Errors, Fraud, and Abuse*, by Holly Stockdale

Financing

- CRS Report RS20173, *Medicare: Financing the Part A Hospital Insurance Program*, by Jennifer O'Sullivan
- CRS Report RS20946, *Medicare: History of Part A Trust Fund Insolvency Projections*, by Jennifer O'Sullivan
- CRS Report RL32582, *Medicare: Part B Premiums*, by Jennifer O'Sullivan
- CRS Report RS21731, *Medicare: Part B Premium Penalty*, by Jennifer O'Sullivan
- CRS Report RS22796, *Medicare Trigger*, by Hinda Chaikind and Christopher M. Davis
- CRS Report RL34407, *The President's Proposed Legislative Response to the Medicare Funding Warning*, by Hinda Chaikind, Jim Hahn, Jennifer O'Sullivan, and Henry Cohen

Part A Issues

- CRS Report RS22399, *Recent Developments in Medicare Affecting Long-Term Care Hospitals*, by Sibyl Tilson
- CRS Report RL32640, *Medicare Payment Issues Affecting Inpatient Rehabilitation Facilities (IRFs)*, by Sibyl Tilson
- CRS Report RL33921, *Medicare's Skilled Nursing Facility Payment*, by Julie Stone
- CRS Report RS22195, *Social Security Disability Insurance (SSDI) and Medicare: The 24-Month Waiting Period for SSDI Beneficiaries Under Age 65*, by Scott Szymendera

Part B Issues

- CRS Report RL31199, *Medicare: Payments to Physicians*, by Jennifer O'Sullivan
- CRS Report RL31419, *Medicare: Payments for Covered Part B Prescription Drugs*, by Jennifer O'Sullivan
- CRS Report RS22769, *Medicare Clinical Laboratories Competitive Bidding Demonstration*, by Barbara English

Medicare Advantage

- CRS Report RL34151, *Private Fee for Service (PFFS) Plans: How They Differ from Other Medicare Advantage Plans*, by Paulette C. Morgan, Hinda Chaikind, and Holly Stockdale
- CRS Report RL32618, *Medicare Advantage Payments*, by Hinda Chaikind and Paulette C. Morgan

Part D Prescription Drug Program

- CRS Report RL34280, *Medicare Part D Prescription Drug Benefit: A Primer*, by Jennifer O'Sullivan
- CRS Report RL33782, *Federal Drug Price Negotiation: Implications for Medicare Part D*, by Jim Hahn
- CRS Report RL33802, *Pharmaceutical Costs: A Comparison of Department of Veterans Affairs (VA)*, Medicaid, and Medicare Policies, by Gretchen A. Jacobson, Sidath Viranga Panangala, and Jean Hearne

End Notes

[1] Department of Health and Human Services, Budget in Brief, 2009 [http://www.hhs.gov/budget/09budget/2009 BudgetInBrief.pdf].
[2] Congressional Budget Office (CBO), Medicare March 2008 Fact Sheet.
[3] CBO, An Analysis of the President's Budgetary Proposals for Fiscal Year 2009 [http://www.cbo.gov/ftpdocs/ 89xx/doc8990/03-19-AnalPresBudget.pdf] and Medicare March 2008 Fact Sheet.
[4] [http://www.cms.hhs.gov/NationalHealthExpendData/Downloads/proj2007.pdf]

CHAPTER SOURCES

The following chapters have been previously published:

Chapter 1 – This is an edited, excerpted and augmented edition of a United States Congressional Budget Office, Background Paper, dated July 2007.

Chapter 2 – This is an edited, excerpted and augmented edition of a United States Congressional Budget Office Background Paper, dated June 2007.

Chapter 3 – These remarks were delivered as Statement of Mark E. Miller, Ph.D., Exective Director, Medicare Payment Advisory Commission, before the subcommittee on Health Committee on Energy and Commerce, U.S. House of Representatives, dated April 18, 2007.

Chapter 4 - This is an edited, excerpted and augmented edition of a United States Congressional Research Service publication, Report Order Code RL33712, dated August 1, 2008.

INDEX

A

accountability, 64
accounting, 33, 36, 37, 42, 44, 46, 48, 49, 96
accuracy, 28, 54, 57, 58
adjustment, 28, 31, 34, 35, 49, 50, 66, 84, 86, 87, 91
adults, 62
age, 9, 22, 34, 50, 70, 77, 78, 81, 85
aggregation, 43
aging, vii, xi, 70
alternative, 40, 59, 71, 85, 95, 96
ambiguity, 5
amyotrophic lateral sclerosis, 77
anemia, 83
annual rate, x, 53
anticancer drug, 83
appendix, 17, 38, 46, 49
apples, 54
assessment, 4, 5, 82, 87
assets, 98
assignment, 80, 86, 89
assumptions, 41, 58, 98
asymptomatic, 81
authority, 92, 93
availability, 3, 4, 77, 91

B

baby boomers, 70
bankruptcy, 5, 76
base rate, vii, 1, 5, 90
base year, 7, 8, 10, 22, 33, 36, 37, 42, 44, 46, 48
behavior, 3, 4, 21, 31, 42, 43, 44

benchmarks, 59, 60, 63, 93
bias, 15, 23, 62
blood, 81
brachytherapy, 89

C

cancer, 81, 89
cancer screening, 81
candidates, 58
capsule, 71
cardiologist, 64, 65
carrier, 34, 49, 50
cataract, 82
category a, 73, 86
cell, 22
certificate, 82
chemotherapy, 83
children, 89
cholesterol, 81
classification, 84, 89
codes, 39, 49, 50, 87
coding, 58
colonoscopy, 81
colorectal cancer, 38
communication, 65
community, x, 53
comorbidity, 84, 85
competition, 55, 91, 101
complement, 55
complexity, 16, 49, 64
compliance, 65, 85
complications, 49, 63
components, 26, 28, 30, 31, 34, 35, 36, 44, 49, 50, 84, 93, 102
composition, 38, 50
computing, 34

concentration, 22
confidence, 42, 64, 65
confidence interval, 42
Congressional Budget Office, 1, 6, 10, 12, 13, 14,
    17, 18, 20, 21, 25, 30, 33, 36, 37, 41, 42, 44,
    46, 47, 48, 49, 65, 70, 102, 103, 107, 109
consensus, vii, xi, 70, 101
consumer price index, 18, 20, 22, 49
consumers, 18, 20, 22
consumption, 4
control, ix, x, xi, 7, 8, 22, 25, 27, 29, 30, 32, 49,
    56, 69, 76
conversion, ix, 25, 27, 28, 29, 30, 31, 32, 33, 34,
    35, 36, 37, 44, 45, 49, 50, 87, 89
cost saving, 66
costs, vii, viii, ix, xi, 1, 5, 6, 25, 27, 28, 29, 32,
    37, 40, 44, 49, 54, 55, 56, 59, 60, 61, 62, 66,
    67, 69, 70, 73, 74, 76, 83, 84, 85, 86, 87, 90,
    91, 94, 95, 96, 97, 98, 99, 100, 101
counseling, 82
counterbalance, 63
couples, 74, 97
covering, 94
cycling, 90

D

data availability, 51
data collection, 63
data set, 7, 9, 10, 34
death, 34, 50
decision-making process, 61
decisions, 55, 61, 67
decomposition, 33, 34, 35, 38, 45, 50, 51
deduction, xi, 69, 70
definition, 92
delivery, vii, xi, 55, 58, 60, 70, 101
demographic change, 38, 50
demographic characteristics, 34, 38, 50
demographic data, 34
demographics, 7, 22
dentures, 99
Department of Health and Human Services, 32,
    50, 96, 103, 104, 107
dependent variable, 8, 14, 17, 43
detection, 50
diabetes, 58, 82
dialysis, 63, 78, 83, 90
diet, 82
diffusion, 58
direct cost, 85
direct costs, 85
disability, 72, 77

discharges, 66
distribution, 6, 8, 10, 12, 13, 50
doctors, 76, 92
drug therapy, vii, 1
drugs, 79, 83, 89, 90, 94, 95, 98

E

earnings, 74, 77, 78, 97
economics, 58
elasticity, 41, 51
elderly, 97
employees, 28, 95, 97
employment, 78, 97
end-stage renal disease, 59, 76
enrollment, 9, 39, 46, 49, 50, 59, 60, 78, 81, 92,
    93, 94, 103
enrollment rates, 39
equality, 44
erythropoietin, 59, 83
estimating, 8, 39, 41, 43, 54
examinations, 38
expenditures, ix, x, 20, 25, 29, 30, 45, 49, 59, 60,
    62, 67, 70, 83, 87, 98, 99, 101

F

failure, 67
family, 82, 104
family history, 82
family income, 104
fat, 81
feedback, 63, 64, 65
finance, 59, 60, 74
financial crisis, 54
financial resources, 67
financing, vii, x, xi, 53, 70, 71, 74, 77, 97, 99,
    102
firms, 4, 56
fixed costs, 21
fixed rate, 5
flexibility, 54, 60, 67, 101
flu shot, 81
focusing, 23, 57
fraud, 54, 64, 65, 67, 96
freedom, 66
funding, vii, xi, 56, 60, 70, 75, 97, 99, 100, 101,
    102
funds, 74, 96, 98, 99, 102

G

GDP, x, xi, 30, 53, 69, 70, 101
General Accounting Office, 21
generation, 101
generic drugs, 95
glasses, 83
goods and services, x, 53, 54
government, 20, 21, 22, 29, 62, 73, 84, 93, 95,
    96, 97, 101
government securities, 96
gross domestic product, x, 30, 53
groups, 4, 5, 8, 10, 22, 38, 41, 57, 58, 59, 66, 86,
    88, 89
growth, ix, x, 5, 26, 27, 29, 30, 33, 34, 35, 36, 38,
    40, 42, 45, 49, 53, 54, 55, 56, 57, 59, 60, 70,
    75, 76, 93, 98, 100
growth rate, 29, 70, 75, 98, 100
guidance, 63
guidelines, 58, 63

H

head injury, 30, 49
health, 1, 2, 3, 4, 8, 16, 19, 22, 25, 39, 49, 53, 54,
    55, 56, 57, 58, 60, 61, 63, 66, 67, 69, 70, 71,
    72, 73, 76, 78, 79, 83, 86, 91, 94, 95, 99, 100,
    101
health care, vii, viii, x, xi, 2, 3, 4, 8, 16, 19, 22,
    53, 54, 55, 56, 57, 58, 60, 61, 63, 67, 70, 72,
    76, 99, 100, 101
health care costs, 61
health care sector, 22
health care system, 67
health expenditure, 70
health insurance, xi, 69, 70, 71, 76, 91
health services, 49, 56, 73, 78, 79, 83, 86
health status, 3
hip, 41
hospice, 49, 78, 79, 87, 91
hospitalization, 72
hospitals, 4, 5, 16, 18, 20, 21, 22, 56, 57, 58, 63,
    66, 80, 84, 85, 86, 89, 92, 96
host, 53
hypertension, 64, 65
hypothesis, 51

I

immunosuppressive drugs, 83
implementation, viii, 2, 5, 6, 9, 11, 29, 99, 100

incentives, 54, 55, 57, 58, 60, 61, 63, 64, 65, 66,
    89, 91, 94, 95
inclusion, 59
income, 3, 4, 9, 11, 19, 20, 26, 39, 40, 74, 75, 76,
    77, 78, 84, 85, 94, 95, 97, 98, 99, 100, 104
income tax, 97
independence, 22
independent variable, 17, 23, 43
indicators, 62, 63
indices, 28, 32, 37, 44
indirect effect, 36
industry, 62
inflation, x, 3, 5, 7, 8, 17, 27, 30, 31, 49, 53, 70,
    87, 88
information technology, 66
infrastructure, 66
injuries, 79
insertion, 83
institutional change, 21
institutions, 5
insurance, xi, 28, 50, 69, 76, 99, 100
integrity, 57
interactions, 22
interference, 95
intermediaries, 96
investment, 62

K

kidney, 72, 78, 83, 90

L

labor, 3, 40, 49, 90
language, 79, 80
laws, 76, 77
legislation, xi, 29, 69, 76, 77, 91, 99, 101, 102
leisure, 3, 4, 40
leisure time, 3, 4
lens, 83
life expectancy, 79
life span, vii, xi, 70, 101
lifestyle, 82
lifetime, 72, 78, 79, 81
likelihood, 55
links, 56
location, 8, 9, 85

M

management, xi, 51, 57, 62, 65, 66, 69, 79, 82
manufacturer, 88

market, 5, 6, 9, 12, 13, 18, 20, 22, 38, 39, 57, 63, 64, 85, 91
market share, 85
marketing, 4, 60
marketplace, 56
markets, viii, 2, 8, 19
measurement, 2, 15, 23, 59, 63, 64, 65
measures, vii, viii, x, 1, 2, 8, 9, 15, 19, 22, 29, 44, 49, 53, 55, 61, 62, 63, 67, 87
median, viii, 2, 88, 89, 90
medical care, 38, 67, 70, 87
Medicare Modernization Act (MMA), xi, 49, 69, 71, 75, 77, 88, 91, 94, 95, 96, 97, 99, 100, 101, 102, 105
men, 81
mental health, 79, 80
military, 100
models, 8, 14, 43, 51, 66
money, 62, 84
morning, 53

N

nation, vii, viii, ix, xi, 1, 25, 29, 69, 70, 76
negative relation, 41
network, 92
nursing, vii, viii, 1, 2, 3, 4, 5, 6, 10, 12, 13, 14, 17, 18, 20, 49, 56, 72, 78, 79, 96
nursing care, 5, 79
nutrition, 82

O

objectivity, 30
observations, 23, 50, 51
observed behavior, 45
occult blood, 81
occupational therapy, 5, 79, 80
omission, 51
organ, 82, 83
osteoporosis, 82
outliers, 84, 85, 86, 89
ownership, 22, 88
oxygen, 82, 88

P

parameter, 43, 51
parliamentary procedure, 75, 99, 102
partnership, 62
pathology, 79, 80
patient care, 49

payroll, 72, 74, 75, 76, 77, 96, 97, 98, 99, 102
peer group, 64
peers, 54, 64, 65, 67
percentile, 12
permit, 61, 89
physical therapy, 79, 80
podiatrists, 49, 80
poor, 61, 63, 65, 76, 104
population, vii, xi, 7, 22, 38, 39, 65, 70, 76, 77, 85, 98, 99, 101
positive relation, 41
positive relationship, 41
poverty, 74, 95, 100, 104
power, 63, 82
premiums, x, xi, 28, 53, 60, 69, 70, 71, 74, 75, 77, 78, 96, 97, 98, 99, 100, 102
presbyopia, 83
pressure, 56, 59
price signals, 57
prices, ix, 3, 4, 5, 7, 8, 22, 25, 28, 34, 35, 36, 41, 49, 50, 56, 67, 95
primary data, 11
private sector, xi, 55, 63, 69, 75, 77, 101
productivity, 33, 36, 37, 42, 44, 46, 48, 49, 54, 56, 57
profit, 22, 39, 40, 54, 57
profit margin, 39
profitability, 57, 58
profits, 21, 54, 59, 60
program, vii, viii, ix, x, xi, 7, 25, 26, 27, 28, 29, 33, 34, 49, 53, 55, 56, 59, 60, 61, 62, 63, 64, 65, 66, 67, 69, 70, 71, 75, 76, 77, 79, 80, 81, 82, 83, 88, 91, 93, 94, 95, 96, 97, 98, 99, 100, 101, 102
prostate, 81
prostate specific antigen, 81

Q

quality improvement, 63, 66

R

race, 34, 50
range, 22, 42, 43, 45, 83, 100, 101
real income, 8
reality, 5
reconciliation, xi, 69, 76, 101
redundancy, 66
reforms, 55, 75, 101
regression, 7, 8, 14, 17, 18, 20, 21, 22, 23, 40, 43, 45, 51

regression analysis, 23
regression equation, 22
regulations, 92
rehabilitation, vii, 1, 22, 56, 79, 80
relationship, 50, 55, 56
relative size, 40
resolution, 75, 99, 102
resources, ix, 25, 28, 29, 32, 37, 44, 49, 58, 61, 65, 66
restructuring, 54
returns, 97
revenue, 27, 75, 77, 96, 97, 99, 101, 102
rewards, 65
risk, 55, 58, 73, 81, 82, 91, 94
risk factors, 82
robustness, viii, 2
R-squared, 18, 20
rural areas, 28, 49, 90

S

sales, 89
sample, 34, 35, 38, 50, 51, 64
savings, 20, 56, 59, 60, 62, 66, 88, 91, 94, 101
scores, 64
securities, 96, 97
self-employed, 97
sensitivity, viii, 2, 41
series, 5, 63, 90
service quality, 56
severity, 58, 84
sex, 9, 22, 34, 50
shares, 16
sharing, 3, 33, 36, 37, 39, 40, 42, 44, 46, 48, 49, 50, 71, 73, 74, 79, 80, 81, 82, 83, 93, 94, 95, 99, 100
side effects, 3, 4
sigmoidoscopy, 81
sign, 18, 20, 51
signals, 57, 60
similarity, 89
social security, 53, 76, 77, 97, 98, 99, 101, 106
Social Security Disability Insurance, 106
social services, 79
social workers, 80
spillover effects, 16
stability, 30
stabilization, 61, 94
stakeholders, 62
standard error, 42, 44
standards, 22, 62, 63, 67, 74
statistics, 6, 11, 12, 13, 14, 46
strategies, 63, 65, 66

subsidy, 60, 94, 95, 96
substitutes, 22
substitution, 4, 40, 51
substitution effect, 4, 40
suppliers, 90
supply, viii, 2, 3, 4, 40, 41, 56, 84
support services, 79, 90
survival, 21
sustainability, x, 53, 66
sustainable growth, 53, 87
symmetry, 41, 43, 44, 51
systems, xi, 21, 53, 55, 56, 57, 58, 61, 63, 64, 66, 67, 69, 76, 77, 84

T

targets, ix, x, 25, 31, 32
tax increase, 54
taxation, 98, 99
teaching, 84, 85
technology, vii, xi, 57, 58, 61, 70, 89, 101
terminal illness, 79
terminally ill, 79
therapists, 80, 87
therapy, 79, 80
threshold, 77, 85
time frame, 15, 99
time periods, 7, 15
tissue, 89
total revenue, 21
trade, 3
trade-off, 3
training, 82
transfer of money, 96
transition, 9, 21, 23, 84
transition period, 21
transitions, 22, 66
transparency, 62
transplantation, 90
trust, 74, 75, 76, 96, 97, 98, 102

U

U.S. Treasury, 96
uniform, 6
unions, 95, 96
unit cost, 21, 62
United States, x, 53, 62, 103, 104, 109
updating, 31
urban areas, 28
urbanization, 9, 11

V

values, 22, 23, 31, 43, 50, 57, 65, 87
variability, 57, 62
variables, 7, 8, 11, 18, 20, 22
variation, 6, 12, 22, 50, 55, 67, 91
vector, 8
volatility, 31

W

wage level, 87

wages

wages, 4, 5, 8, 9, 11, 18, 20, 21, 22, 28, 86
watershed, 55
welfare, 76
women, 81
workers, 4, 56, 74, 76

Y

yield, 41, 43